Intermittent Fasting for Beginners

Diana Lor & Anna Watson

© **Copyright 2018 by Diana Lor & Anna Watson**
All rights reserved.

The following Book is reproduced below with the goal of providing information that is as accurate and reliable as possible. Regardless, purchasing this eBook can be seen as consent to the fact that both the publisher and the author of this book are in no way experts on the topics discussed within and that any recommendations or suggestions that are made herein are for entertainment purposes only. Professionals should be consulted as needed prior to undertaking any of the action endorsed herein.

This declaration is deemed fair and valid by both the American Bar Association and the Committee of Publishers Association and is legally binding throughout the United States.

Furthermore, the transmission, duplication, or reproduction of any of the following work including specific information will be considered an illegal act irrespective of if it is done electronically or in print. This extends to creating a secondary or tertiary copy of the work or a recorded copy and is only allowed with the express written consent from the Publisher. All additional rights reserved.

The information in the following pages is broadly considered a truthful and accurate account of facts and as such, any inattention, use, or misuse of the information in question by the reader will render any resulting actions solely under their purview. There are no scenarios in which the publisher or the original author of this work can be in any fashion deemed liable for any hardship or damages that may befall them after undertaking information described herein.

Additionally, the information in the following pages is intended only for informational purposes and should thus be thought of as universal. As befitting its nature, it is presented without assurance regarding its prolonged validity or interim quality. Trademarks that are mentioned are done without written consent and can in no way be considered an endorsement from the trademark holder.

Table of Contents

Introduction 1

The Obesity Epidemic 3

Intermittent Fasting- An Easy Way to Holistic Health 6

    That is it. Your body will do the rest. 6

    The Process 7

    Eat-Stop-Eat Fasts 10

    Alternate Day Fasts 11

Intermittent Fasting for You- The Beginners Dilemma 12

    The Way To Do It 14

    Start By Elimination 17

The Main Cause of Fat Gain - Unhealthy Food and Poor Eating Habits 21

    Unhealthy Food 22

    Poor Eating Habits 23

History of Intermittent Fasting 27

    Case for Fasting 28

    Fasting as a Practice 30

- The practice of Religious Fasting 31
  - Fasting by Muslims During Ramadan 31
  - Benefits of Ramadan Fasting 31
- Intermittent Fasting in Jainism 32
  - Jains are pure vegetarians 32
  - Jains didn't Even Eat Root Vegetables 33
  - Shorter Eating Windows 33

Unsustainability- The Reason Diets Fail You 35

- The difference in the Functioning of Diets and Intermittent Fasting 35
  - Diets Lead to Lower Metabolism 35
  - Diets Lead to Nutrient Deficiency 37
  - Diets are Difficult and Unsustainable 38
  - Diets Lead to Binge Eating 39
- Exercise As a Lone Way to Lose Weight 40

Intermittent Fasting Methods 43

- A Very Important Thing To Do Is To NOT Rush the Process 45
- If you want your intermittent fasting to be successful: 45

Don't Set Ambiguous Goals- Set Easily Achievable Goals 46

Develop a Clear Understanding of the Chosen Intermittent Fasting Method 47

Don't Get Disheartened by the Small Road Bumps 47

The 5:2 Fasts 49

I. The 5 normal eating days 49

II. The 2 fasting days 50

The 12 Hour Fasts 52

The Method 52

The Ways to Make it Work 53

The Impact 54

Meal Management 54

The First Meal 54

The Second Meal 55

The Third Meal 55

The 16:8 Plan- The Lean gain Method 58

The 16:8 Plan for Men 58

The 16:8 Plan for Women 59

The Routine 60

The 16:8 Plan for Morning People 61

The 16:8 Plan for the Night owls 62

It's Simple 62

The 20:4 Intermittent Plan- The Warrior Fasts 66

You Must Keep in Mind the Following Things Before Taking Up 20:4 Intermittent Fasting 69

Some Key Notes for the Success of 20:4 Intermittent Fasting 70

Eat-Stop-Eat Plan 72

Key Tips for Eat-Stop-Eat Intermittent Fasting .. 74

Alternate Day Fasts 76

The Science Behind Intermittent Fasting 79

Why Do We Accumulate Fat? 80

How Intermittent Fasting Helps in Fat Burning? 81

Advantages of Burning Fat 82

How Does It Happen? 82

Intermittent Fasting and Ketosis 84

Fat Burning Element of Intermittent Fasting 86

Functions of Insulin 86

Problems with Poor Reception of Insulin 87

The Process of Insulin Production 88

High Insulin Leads to Fat Accumulation 88

Problems in Fat Burning 89

This is How Intermittent Fasting Helps 89

Problems with Diets and Other Weight Loss Measures 91

Health Benefits of Intermittent Fasting 94

Improving Heart Health 94

Lower Risk of Diabetes 96

Lowers the Risk of Chronic Inflammation 97

Things to Check Before You Begin Intermittent Fasting 100

History of Eating Disorders 101

Diabetes 101

Under Medication 102

Lactating or Pregnant Women 102

People Suffering from Gallbladder Issues 103

People with Unregulated Thyroid 103

Children and Teenagers 104

Tips to Succeed with Your Intermittent Fasting Routine 105

Walks are Good 106

Don't Overstrain Yourself on the Fasting Days 106

Keep Yourself Occupied....................................... 107

Don't Indulge in Emotional Eating 107

Include Healthy Things in Your Diet 108

Drink Non-caloric Beverages to Avoid Hunger Pangs 108

Do not Give in to the Pressure of the Breakfast 108

Choose a Diet That Works the Best for You 109

Remain Positive 109

Foods That Help and the Foods to Avoid 110

Few Important Things to Include are: 110

    Water.. 110

    Fish 111

    Avocado... 111

    Leafy Greens 112

    Potatoes... 113

    Eggs 113

    Whole Grains 113

    Probiotics 114

    Legumes 114

- Nuts 115
- The Foods to Avoid 115
  - Processed Foods 115
  - Junk Foods 116
  - Alcohol 117
  - Juices 117

Key Factors in the Success of Intermittent Fasting 118

- Food 119
- Exercise 122
- Sleep 123
- Routine 125

Important Points to Follow in Intermittent Fasting 127

- Don't Overeat- It Will Only Make Things Difficult for You 127
- Exercise in Fasted State & Even on the Fasting Days 127
- Drink Water and Remain Hydrated 128
- Drinking Unsweetened Black Tea or Coffee is Good 129
- Delay- Shift the First Meal of the Day Farthest 129

Don't Fear Food 130

Common Myths about Intermittent Fasting 131

Myth #1: Morning Breakfast is the Most Important Meal of the Day 131

Myth #2: Fasting will Lead to Muscle Wasting 133

Myth #3: You will Get Weak if You Fast 134

Myth #4: You will have Low Blood Sugar 136

Myth #5: Your Body will Go into Starvation Mode 137

The Best Thing About Intermittent Fasting 139

Easy 140

Effective 141

Convenient 141

Intermittent Fasting is for Everyone 142

Difficult Food Choices 142

Wheat or Gluten Intolerance 143

Lack of Time 143

Financial Constraints 144

People Who are Always on the Move 145

People Who Detest Cooking 145

Elderly 146

It is Possible for Everyone 146

It is Flexible 147

It Gives You Power and Control 147

Conclusion **148**

Introduction

In this book we will discuss the basics of intermittent fasting and the ways in which it can help you. You will get to know the impact of intermittent fasting on various aspects of your health.

Intermittent fasting has emerged as a popular way to lose weight in the past for some time. It has been showing great promise, and people around the world are reaping the benefits of this easy to follow weight loss measure.

The best thing about intermittent fasting is the ease with which it can be made a part of life. You can follow it irrespective of the type of job you do or profession you follow. It is simple, yet very effective.

Intermittent fasting can make you lose weight very fast. But, that's only one benefit of incorporating intermittent fasting in your lifestyle. It brings to you a number of other health benefits too. You will feel healthier, more energetic, and lively. It has strong anti-aging benefits and also improves the health of your heart and other organs.

However, in over enthusiasm people misinterpret the whole principle of intermittent fasting. It isn't a fat diet. It isn't simply a way to lose fat. It is a complete lifestyle change. It is a way of life you can follow without any difficulty throughout your whole life and still be healthy. Understanding this subtle difference in detail can make a world of difference.

This book is an attempt to bring all the aspects of intermittent fasting in front of you. This book will enlighten you about the ways in which you can make intermittent fasting a way of your life.

It will show you the right way to follow this wonderful routine and bring positivity in your life. You will also get to know all the details of the process and the challenges you might face in the way.

This book has tried to explain the nitty-gritty of the process to clear things completely.

In this book, you will find the ways you can benefit from intermittent fasting the most, and lose a lot of weight and belly fat fast. It will give you the keys to success and the important things to keep in mind while following an intermittent fasting routine.

Chapter 1

THE OBESITY EPIDEMIC

We live in a world of facts and figures. We waste no time in rubbishing claims that are unsubstantiated by facts. When we have facts in front of us, we work to improve. Humanity has thrived this way for thousands of years.

Humankind has never been the strongest, the bravest, the fastest, or the biggest race. Several other species on earth have that honor. Yet, humankind is still leading the race. It has only been possible because we have been able to learn from our mistakes and improve. We never submitted to the shortcomings. We rose above the circumstances and thrived.

However, it is astonishing that we are ignoring or undermining the dangers of obesity so easily. Obesity is one of the 5 major causes of preventable deaths all over the world. In fact, obesity and related disorders lead to more than 400,000 preventable deaths every year in the US alone. It is simply not just a cosmetic problem. It does much more than making us look bad. Obesity brings with itself heart diseases, diabetes, cholesterol, and other metabolic disorders.

The obesity epidemic is at our doors. It is a global pandemic. WHO report of 2016 says that over 40% of the world population is overweight. Over 13% of the global population is obese and the problem is escalating really fast. The global obesity rates have tripled since 1975.

The obesity problem in the US and Europe is even steeper. The Center for Disease Control and Prevention (CDC) reports say that more than 70% of Americans adults are battling excess weight issues. This is not all, 39.6% of the US adult population is actually obese.

Obesity is a problem that is getting out of control. Obesity is not a lone rider. It attacks like a pack of wolves. A number of other problems arise with obesity. They seize the victims and make recovery difficult. Obesity is a problem we can't ignore.

However, the larger problem is that we have been trying to overpower the obesity epidemic and have failed successively. Obesity is not a latent problem like blood pressure or cholesterol. When a person gets obese, it is visible. People have been trying to control their weight but most of the weight control measures have failed them. Diets, pills, exercise, and other measures show some results initially, but the weight comes back. There has been no way to control weight in the long run.

Intermittent Fasting has emerged as a savior. It is a fast, easy, and reliable way to lose weight and remain healthy. You can follow intermittent fasting irrespective of your social, financial or work conditions. It is viable for you even if you don't have time. It works for you even if you can't do much physical exercise. The best thing of all, it costs you NOTHING.

Intermittent fasting is an easy way to get rid of most health issues. But you can easily overcome most of your health issues by following an easy and simple routine.

If this sounds interesting, this book will be a revelation for you!

Chapter 2

INTERMITTENT FASTING- AN EASY WAY TO HOLISTIC HEALTH

Intermittent fasting is no magic wand, but its effect is magical indeed.

Intermittent fasting is a way of keeping short fasts to remain healthy. There is no magic trick involved. You do not need to know many things to practice intermittent fasting. To begin with, this is a way to give your body, the time to process the food. You can follow intermittent fasting simply by remaining in a fasted state for a specific number of hours in a day.

That is it. Your body will do the rest.

However, your mind will need an explanation. It is unwise to trust things without knowing them. Let us start with the process first and then we'll discuss the way it affects your body.

The Process

You will have to follow specific eating and fasting hours in a day. Let's call each feasting and fasting session as a window. Therefore, intermittent fasting is the process of having short feasting windows and long fasting windows. There will be no dieting or calorie restriction and yet, you'll be able to lose weight and belly fat.

The whole weight loss impact lies in maintaining strict fasting windows. Managing these windows isn't a difficult job as you only need to extend your fasting state for a few hours every day.

Let's say you follow a standard routine and have a regular job.

- You leave to go to the office around 8 or 9 in the morning. Most people have their breakfast a few minutes before they leave.
- The eating day starts around 8 or 9 am.
- You have the morning snacks around 11 am.
- You do your lunch before 2 pm.
- You have tea and snacks around 4 pm.

- You leave the office and have a bite on your way. This puts an evening snack around 6 pm.
- This gives you another 2 hours for dinner and you usually have your dinner around 8 or 9 pm.

This is a basic eating routine for most people. The morning birds wake up a bit early and can feel the urge to eat one or two hours early. In that case, you will also have to take into account the fact that they would also be sleeping early. So, you can accordingly shift their dinner timing. Even if you are a night bird, your morning schedule automatically shifts a bit farther. It makes little difference to your feasting and fasting hours in a day.

The fact of the matter is that we usually have 12-14 hours of feasting and fasting schedule. This has been going on for years as a habit as most of us feel neither anything odd nor uncomfortable about this.

You actually follow 10-12 hours of fast daily. You can begin intermittent fasting by extending the fasting windows by a couple more hours. It isn't a very difficult task at all. You don't need a lot of grit, determination, willpower or other such attributes.

You only have to refrain eating for a few more hours in a day.

However, things can look pretty easy on paper and become difficult in practice. Simply extending the fasting window by 4 hours can be a lot to ask. You may feel that staying hungry for a few more hours is not much. But, believe me, it is.

Not doing something is bad, but doing it without any preparation is pathetic and this is how you'll feel if you aren't prepared. This book will help you with the preparation that you need. You will be able to keep the fasts with great control.

Intermittent Fasting is the process of staying hungry for a greater number of hours in a day than you eat. There are several ways to keep intermittent fasts like:

5:2 Fasts

This is the easiest intermittent fasting schedule to follow. You only need to fast on any two days of the week and you can eat responsibly in the rest of the five days. On your fasting days, you will need to limit your calorie intake. For women, the calorie limit is 500 and for men, it is 600. You can have 2-3 meals even on the fasting days but you will have to ensure that you remain in the calorie range.

16:8 Fasts

This is one of the most commonly followed intermittent fasting practice. You need to stay in the fasting state for 16 hours in a day and eat in the remaining 8 hours. It is easy to follow in daily routine.

20:4 Fasts

This is the warrior fast. You get 4 hours of eating window and have to remain in the fasting state for 20 hours in a day. It is a bit tough as you get to have only one meal in a day. But, it yields great results. It is one of the most favorite ways for bodybuilders.

Eat-Stop-Eat Fasts

This fast raises the difficulty level of the routine. In this fast, you have to remain in the fasted state for the complete 24-hour duration. You can eat responsibly on the non-fasting days. You can keep up to 2 such fasts in a week.

Alternate Day Fasts

The concept is the same as eat-stop-eat. You only need to keep them every alternate day. These are difficult, as staying hungry regularly sometimes gets tough.

These are some of the intermittent fasting schedules for beginners and we will discuss them in detail in the upcoming chapters.

The most difficult part of intermittent fasting is to take the plunge and begin. People keep postponing and putting off the idea and often never start. Intermittent fasting is a very easy and effective way to manage weight and other health issues.

In the next chapter, we will discuss the ways we can make intermittent fasting easy and possible.

Chapter 3

Intermittent Fasting for You- The Beginners Dilemma

Beginning something is the biggest part of the problem. The first step is the hardest to take. We make plans to do things and then we postpone them to the next day. We all very well know that tomorrow never comes.

Food is important. We all love food. The struggle of mankind started with food and we still continue to fight for food. We spend a big part of our earnings on food, even today. The idea of staying away from food is bound to sound intimidating. There is nothing to be coy about it. In fact, admitting your fears is the best way to face them.

If you are worried that you may not be able to fast for 16, 20 or 24 hours, you are absolutely right. But, you don't even have to. Beginning of anything should always be on a strong footing and then only the things can last. Fasting is no different. If you have recently started considering the idea of intermittent fasting for managing your weight or other health issues, then diving straight with the long fasts will be a bad idea. This argument has valid reasons.

Reasons for not to begin with long fasts:

- ➢ If you have been exploiting food, your body is accustomed to having food at short intervals. The temptation of food will make your life difficult. You are more likely to leave the routine abruptly and that will be bad.
- ➢ Your stomach doesn't release the hormones that make you feel on the basis of need for food. It releases them on the basis of your eating routine. It may come at a surprise but try to rethink it. You always start feeling hungry around the same time daily.
- ➢ Your body needs time to adjust to every change. Fasting is a big change as it involves several crucial processes in your body. Subjecting your body to such big changes all of a sudden, will put it under a lot of

pressure. You must ensure that you always switch slowly to any kind of change, good or bad.

The Way To Do It

Your first step towards intermittent fasting and good health is to control meal frequency. For the moment, stop worrying about the calories, kind of food or any other such thing. The number of meals we have in a day is enough to destroy our health.

Food gives our body the required energy. However, we only need a limited amount of energy to survive. The rest of the food simply gets stored as fat. But, it is not the bone of contention at the moment.

Suppose you have an electrical appliance. The best one in the market that has been ever produced. It has no manufacturing errors. It can work great. But, would you keep running it forever. Every machine needs rest. Excess of anything is bad. We are doing the same to our body with frequent meals.

Our body is the best engineering marvel in this world. Even with the current level of advancement of science and technology we cannot replicate it.

However, we cannot subject it to overuse and we are doing the same by eating frequently.

- Our body takes around 8 to 12 hours to process the food we eat. It is a lengthy process.
- When you eat something your digestion process gets to work.
- It transforms the food into glucose and sends it into your bloodstream.
- This raises your blood sugar levels.
- Your pancreas senses the high level of blood sugar and releases insulin to help the cells absorb the glucose for energy.
- Insulin helps the cells in absorbing glucose.
- The cells can only use a limited amount of glucose.
- The insulin then stores the extra glucose as glycogen in muscles and liver. The limit for storage of glucose as glycogen is also low.
- The remaining glucose is stored as fat in your body.
- This is a slow process. You can't rush your body.

Your body has to run this process all over again with every meal you take. Even if it is small or big meal. Even eating cookies also go through the same process.

This means, if you snack frequently, your digestion and fat storage process will never be at rest. There is no way you are going to get slim this way.

The first step in getting a slimmer body, is to put a control on frequent snacking and having meals at short intervals.

It will help you in several ways:

i. It will help you in getting habitual of staying away from food
ii. Your calorie intake will definitely go down. We don't realize but even small snacks also add a lot of calories. You have got to admit the fact that you are not eating broccoli and spinach in snacks. snacks are unhealthy and fattening.
iii. The longer you maintain the interval between meals, the better for your digestive system.

Start By Elimination

The best and the simplest way to begin is to eliminate snacks from your routine. It is the key to success. Normally, we at least 6 meals a day including the snacks. Some people may be having more if they are in a habit of eating chocolates, candies or other such things. Remember, anything that adds calories is a meal for your body.

Therefore, your target should be to eliminate the snacks and stick to main meals.

The best way to do this is to avoid eating apart from 3 meals a day.

- Have a healthy and nutritious breakfast in the morning.
- Include healthy fat, proteins, and fiber-rich food in your breakfast.
- Avoid sugar or syrups. Sugar induces cravings. The more sugar you have in your food, the faster you will feel the cravings to eat.
- The more protein and fat you'll have, the less eager you'll feel to eat snacks. They give you

a feeling of satiety and you don't feel like eating.

If you are worried about eating fat, you should stop worrying about it at the moment. Eating fat is not the cause of obesity and we will get to that later in the book.

A healthy and heavy breakfast will help you feel satisfied until lunchtime. You are unlikely to feel hungry for snacks.

But, if you do feel the urge, stick to unsweetened beverages like fresh lime water, black coffee or black tea. Do not go on the road that takes you to sweetened beverages like sodas, energy drinks, or anything else that adds calories to your system. The point here is not to restrict the number of calories, but to ensure that your digestive system works smooth.

Try to keep all your meals healthy and nutritious. Include all the macronutrients like carbohydrates, fats, and protein in good proportions. A balance of these nutrients induces satiety. It will help in staying away from snacks easy. If you feel the urge, you can have unsweetened beverages. Try to stay away from sweets, processed food, and junk food as much as possible.

If you stick to this routine for a few days, you will be able to bring yourself to 3 meals a day. It is no mean feat. The day you are able to avoid all types of snacks and sustain easily on 3 main meals in the day, give yourself a pat on the back. You have cleared the first hurdle.

This point forward, the only task at hand is to shift your breakfast a little towards your lunch. You should also start shifting the lunch towards the dinner. The aim should always be to limit all the 3 meals at least in an 8 hour period.

This will and should take time. The longer you take to reach and the steady you remain, the higher will be your chances of success.

If you stick to the plan and remain consistent, intermittent fasting will become easy for you. Staying hungry for a few hours is not a difficult task at all. We are not energy deprived. Most of us are leading a sedentary lifestyle. Our calorie expenditure is low but we consume more than that. This energy gets stored as fat.

The next step is to have healthy eating habits.

Intermittent fasting doesn't force you to limit your calorie intake. You can eat the things that you like. However, eating unhealthy things or having unhealthy eating habits have a negative impact on our health. It slows the process of getting good results.

You can speed up the process of fat burning and amplify the impact of intermittent fasting by adopting healthy eating habits. It will also help you in remaining consistent in your approach.

The next chapter will throw some light on the unhealthy foods we consume and the poor eating habits we follow. It will help you in understanding their impact on your health.

Chapter 4

The Main Cause of Fat Gain - Unhealthy Food and Poor Eating Habits

It would be honest, to begin with, a disclaimer. Unhealthy food and poor eating habits are not the only cause of obesity. Genetics and hormonal issues can cause obesity. Side effects of medications and prolonged sickness can also lead to obesity.

However, it would remain an undisputed fact that unhealthy food and poor eating choices are the biggest cause of obesity. You can't really expect to have the carved body of Adonis by eating junk food. Hercules did not get all that power and fame by eating French fries and chips.

Unhealthy food and poor eating habits have been two major reasons for the health debacle. We have ignored the importance of both these aspects and taken them for granted. It has not fared well for us.

Unhealthy Food

We live in a fast-paced world. The neck-breaking speed of life has made it convenient to eat fast food. It comes cheap and without costing time. However, one fact that we conveniently ignore is that this food not only comes cheap, but it is cheap. It doesn't matter the kind of quality a fast-food chain boasts. The fact that it is fast makes it bad. You can't expect the vegetable oil which is being heated the whole day to give you anything else besides cancer. No one in the sane mind would expect loads of sauces and sugars in fast food to add to good health. The endless barraging of sodas will not bring good health. These food items can only make you fat. The more you'll eat them, the unhealthier you'll become.

Fast food lovers believe that there is a widespread prejudice against this kind of food but there is none. The deteriorating health of people, in general, is a live testimony.

- Medical science has proven it beyond doubt that fried food is unhealthy and most of fast food is fried.
- It has also been proven without a doubt that sugar-laced food is bad for your health and

leads to weight gain. Sugar is the main component of most of the fast foods.
- Most of the fat-free foods have a lot of added sugar to add taste to the food. Sugar is addictive and causes cravings.
- Sugar also adds empty calories to your system that makes you fat and does not give anything good to your digestive system.
- Sodas, alcohol, energy drinks, and other aerated sweetened beverages are also not helping the cause. They are also increasing obesity.

Poor Eating Habits

Eating habits play a very important role in our health. They are crucial for proper digestion of the food so that the body can function optimally.

Some of the good habits that we learn at a young age:

- We must eat slowly
- We must chew the food properly
- Eating all the vegetables is important
- We must not talk while eating
- No TV while eating
- No Mobile Phones while eating

However, soon enough we forget most of these and get on the way of spoiling our health. All these habits have a role to play in our health.

We must eat slowly: Eating slowly helps in making us feel fuller sooner. Our body takes some time to realize that we have eaten the required amount. If we eat fast, the body is not able to convey the signal and you tend to overeat.

We must chew the food properly: Proper chewing of the food helps in better digestion. If you chew your food properly, eating gets slow and you consume less food. Therefore, effectively it helps in preventing the chances of overeating.

Finishing the vegetables: Vegetables are important. They are full of vitamins and minerals. They are essential for your body. However, there is one very important aspect of eating vegetables. They help in the aid of preventing you from getting fat. Yes, the vegetables, especially the non-starchy leafy greens have negligible calories and lots of fiber and nutrients. They help you feel full very fast. You can eat them as much as you like without worries.

We must NOT talk while eating: Talking, discussing things, or sharing stories is a fun way to have meals. But unfortunately, it is not the healthy way. You lose track of the amount of food that can go inside you while you have a light banter and socialize at the dinner table. Eating mindfully is a very important thing. Overeating is not going to help you in any way.

NO TV while eating: The reason is the same as talking while eating. You are so immersed in the information overload that you pay no focus to the amount of food that goes inside you.

ABSOLUTELY NO Smartphones while eating: The reasons are again clear. They divert your attention from food and you either overeat or don't eat enough. Both the cases are bad for your health.

These are simple eating rules that we defy and overlook on a regular basis which have an impact on our health. However, the biggest mistake is the habits of frequent snacking. It has the most serious consequences. It is a habit that suits us as well and the food producers and therefore, we will want to stick to it.

The key to stay fit and reduce the belly fat is to improve your eating habits. Ignoring these key rules will make it hard for you to stick to the routine. These are simple rules that we can follow to stay fit and healthy.

You can get unimaginable results if you stick to a healthy eating routine and follow intermittent fasting. It is a sure shot way of regaining health and becoming fit. Intermittent fasting is not some fad diet. In fact, it isn't a diet at all. It is a lifestyle that helps you in becoming fit and healthy. It is a sustainable way to live your life. It can easily become a part of your life and you can follow it in the normal course of life.

The following chapter will shed some light of the way intermittent fasting has been a part of our lives for thousands of years. It will also discuss the ways in which people still follow it and really benefit from it a lot.

Chapter 5

History of Intermittent Fasting

Intermittent fasting has always been a part of our lifestyle. Our ancestors started their journey on this earth as hunter-gatherers. They had few means to survive and they were completely dependent on nature for food. They either gathered food from trees or had to hunt. They had little control over the outcome of both these activities.

Food from trees was seasonal. The wild beasts were difficult to catch. We were never the strongest, fastest and the biggest of the race. Hence, our ancestors were not always lucky to have food whenever they aspired. The periods of feasts and famines were frequent. Our ancestors feasted all they could when they had food and fasted the rest of the time, as they had no way to preserve or store the food for long. This made intermittent fasting as a way of life for them. One thing you can be sure that our ancestors battled a lot less with the menace of obesity than us.

Case for Fasting

People have the misconception that they will face weakness, fatigue or other problems if they fast. If you also have the same fears that your worries are misplaced. The human body has passed through thousands of years of evolution. It is designed to survive even in the worst conditions and fasting for short periods is least of its concerns. Our body has a due process to store energy for later use. The fat in your body is the energy store. It is the insurance policy of your body to survive even in long periods of food deprivations.

Whenever you eat something, your body can utilize only a limited amount of the energy extracted from the food. Your body converts the rest of energy into fat. This fat serves many functions in your body. All the hormones are made from fat. Your body uses the fat for thermostatic functions. However, excess fat is not good for your body. It was never designed to withstand an excess of anything.

The modern age has brought food security and has also led to easy access to food. We added taste to the food and made it a luxury. This has led to the big problem of obesity.

If you believe that remaining in the fasted state will make you weak or impair your abilities to work, then you have never been more incorrect. Our ancestors had no security of food. They went through long periods of deprivation. When they went without food, they needed to be sharper and faster in order to get food. They had to catch the faster and stronger animals. If they couldn't function well, they would have perished in that condition. In the fasted state, your cognitive functions become even sharper. You are able to think fast and memorize better. It is the way of the body to make itself more useful and survive. In fact, recent studies have concluded that intermittent fasting can have a very positive impact on neurodegenerative disorders like Alzheimer's and Parkinson's disease.

In the fasted state, your body starts using the fat as the source of energy. Fat is a clean source of fuel for your body and it gives more energy. In the initial days of fasting, you may feel a bit of weakness as your body is not accustomed to using fat as an energy source. You have exploited it by providing a ready and excessive supply of carbohydrate energy. It is easy to burn and doesn't force the body to use its fat reserves. However, when you remain in the fasted state, your body has no other option than to burn fat for energy. The initial adjustment takes a couple of days but afterward, you'll feel more energetic and lively in the fasted state. There is no reason for you to worry about feeling weak, dull, or lazy during your fasts. This situation will change very soon for good.

Fasting as a Practice

Fasting has been in practice in various cultures. There are several religious practices that require fasting. Most of the fasts practiced are short and hence their impact cannot be measured. However, there are two strong cases of fasting in religious practices that have shown their impact.

The practice of Religious Fasting

Fasting by Muslims During Ramadan

Muslims observe fasting in the month of Ramadan for a considerable period of time. They begin their fast early in the morning before sunrise around 4 am. They break their fast in the evening after sundown around 6 pm. This gives them around 14 hours of fast. During this period they do not eat anything. They are prohibited even to drink water in the fasting period.

Benefits of Ramadan Fasting

- Improvement in HDL (Good Cholesterol)
- Reduction of LDL (Bad Cholesterol)
- Improved Insulin Sensitivity
- Improvement in Blood Sugar levels
- It helps in detoxification
- It helps in appetite reduction
- Your body develops the ability to absorb more nutrients

Intermittent Fasting in Jainism

Jainism is a religion followed in India. Its history goes back to thousands of years. However, the important thing to note is the way intermittent fasting is incorporated in the religion and its impact. The followers of Jainism specifically belong to the business community. Jains have been traditional traders. Their profession required a more sedentary lifestyle even at the time when people relied more on manual labor. Thousands of years ago too, Jains were not the cultivators or craftsmen, they were traders. They had shops and businesses. This meant that they spent most of their time sitting in one place. To avoid the menace of obesity, the religious heads developed a way of life that led to intermittent fasting.

You need to understand a few important things about Jains for understanding how well they have used food to their benefit.

Jains are pure vegetarians

They didn't need to do hard labor. This meant that their protein requirements were low. They didn't need to digest complex foods to survive.

Vegetarianism as a way of life helped them a lot. Most of the high energy difficult to digest food items got eliminated from their diet in one stroke.

Jains didn't Even Eat Root Vegetables

Root vegetables are starchy and have high sugar and carbohydrate content. This could make them fat. They were prohibited from eating them.

Shorter Eating Windows

One of the main principles of Jainism is to eat before sundown. Jains traditionally didn't eat after sundown. It is a highly religious community and hence the morning rituals are long. They get to eat only after finishing their morning rituals and that even shifts their breakfast time. It means they get a limited window to eat in the day.

This community has been following intermittent fasting ingrained into its culture. It has benefitted a lot. It had been a healthy lifestyle that had helped them in staying fit in absence of physical labour or gyms.

You can see that intermittent fasting is not a new practice. Humankind has been following it for thousands of years, knowingly or unknowingly. It has helped us in staying fit and healthy.

Even today you can get the same benefits if you change your lifestyle up a bit. Intermittent fasting will help you in shedding lots of belly fat and weight. You will feel more energetic and thwart away many health issues that come in a package deal with obesity.

Following intermittent fasting is not at all difficult. In fact, it becomes a part of your lifestyle so easily that you don't have to put any effort into following it. This makes it a more sustainable way of losing weight and belly fat. This is also one of the main reasons it is so much better and effective than dieting and other weight loss measures.

In the following chapter, we will discuss the reasons dieting and other weight loss measures fail us. It will also highlight the reasons intermittent fasting triumphs.

Chapter 6

UNSUSTAINABILITY- THE REASON DIETS FAIL YOU

It is a well-acknowledged fact that if you want to lose weight, you will have to reduce the calorie intake. The math is very simple. If the number of calories you consume is higher than the number of calories you burn, you will simply gain fat. The diets of all kinds have been trying to bank exclusively on this principle. But, then why do they fail?

If you look closely, the diets don't suit our bodies. They cause more harm to our bodies than they can help.

The difference in the Functioning of Diets and Intermittent Fasting

Diets Lead to Lower Metabolism

Diets create a temporary shortage of energy. However, they are only focusing on reducing the calorie intake. But, you can't trick your body into failing. When you reduce the calorie intake, your body senses that something is wrong. It maps the shortfall and starts adjusting itself to cope with the calorie deficit. This means that if you start consuming a fewer number of calories, then your body will slow the rate of burning of calories. This is one of the reasons you feel low on diets. Your body lowers the metabolism to cope with the shortage. So, in reality, you are not burning your fat. Your body has evolved to survive. If it feels that the energy supply is low, it will not start burning the energy reserves mindlessly, it will conserve them. The best way to do so is to reduce energy consumption. So, losing fat on diets becomes difficult. You have to get to really severe calorie restrictive diets to force your body to burn fat. However, it adjusts the metabolic rate, and you end up not losing weight. This is among the prime reasons for weight loss getting plateaued for people on diets. They need to make adjustments very often.

Intermittent fasting works in an entirely different way. It doesn't create a shortfall. You eat healthy amounts of food in your eating windows. This always gives a signal that there is no energy deficit.

The fasting windows create a temporary energy demand for the body. It knows that energy supply is in abundance and therefore feels no risk in using the energy stores.

Diets Lead to Nutrient Deficiency

Another big problem with diets is that they lead to nutrient deficiencies. The way of diets is to restrict the calorie intake, this means you need to lower the number of calories you can consume. It leads to a restriction on eating most of the food products. Your reliance on low carbohydrate and low-fat foods increases. One important thing to understand here is that all the macronutrients are important. They have important roles to play in the functioning of our body. Whole grains, for instance, are a source of carbohydrate, but, they also provide you with fiber and various trace minerals. Without the intake of trace minerals, proper functioning of the body gets affected. Fat is an important part of our food, even in small quantities it gives us a lot of energy. It is the base for forming hormones, cell structure, and other important things. Your body cannot function properly without the fat intake. This is among the prime reasons that diets make you feel drained, weak, and lethargic.

Intermittent fasting puts no restriction on food to eat. In fact, you must eat a healthy mix of all the macronutrients while you follow intermittent fasting. It helps you stay in the fasted state without discomfort, keeping you feeling more energetic and strong.

Diets are Difficult and Unsustainable

This is a no-brainer. Diets are depriving and that makes them difficult. The longer you have to forcibly suppress the desire to eat something, the stronger and difficult the feeling gets. This one fact usually makes diets unmanageable. There is a whole world of food items that you like but you can't eat because you are on a diet. It leads to temptation. Suppressing the temptation to eat things leads to irritation and mood swings. Some people also start facing depression due to dieting, which can make people restless and long for the diets to end. The motivation simply remains to lose some weight. You cannot remain on diets for very long and there are several reasons for that. The biggest reason is that diets stop showing the results after some time, and the weight begins to plateau eventually.

Intermittent fasting, on the other hand, is a lifestyle change. Once you accept it, there is no discomfort. You don't need to restrain yourself from eating anything. You can eat anything in small quantities. Unhealthy food is bad, but you can still have fast food with your friends and family if you have to. It becomes a part of your life and doesn't ask you to do something out of the ordinary. This enables you to follow it in a normal fashion and causes no obstruction. You feel no temptation to change anything as there is no resistance, and your body quickly adapts to the change in schedule caused by intermittent fasting. Your hunger pangs subside, and you stop feeling hungry at irregular timings which make you feel more content. This makes intermittent fasting a very sustainable way to lose weight.

Diets Lead to Binge Eating

One of the biggest disadvantages of diets is that they lead to binge eating once you get off the diet. You have been wanting to eat so many things when you were on a diet, but couldn't eat that it becomes difficult to control. People usually get off diets and start binge eating not long after. Low and behold, they end up gaining more weight than they had actually lost. Reports say that at least 80% of the people who lose weight through dieting regain the weight within a matter of a few months or over the course of a few years. Weight loss through this measure is not sustainable. The biggest reason for the fallout is the unsustainability of the process.

Intermittent fasting is an easily sustainable method to live by. Cases of several religions and practices are a live testimony that you can follow intermittent fasting for the whole of your life without any difficulty. This factor makes it the best way to lose weight.

Exercise As a Lone Way to Lose Weight

There are other measures to lose weight like exercise. It is a good way to burn calories and a must for everyone. However, if you are already obese, exercise is a very difficult way to lose weight and most obese people are not able to stick to the routine. Everyone is not cut out for that kind of hard work.

Regular high-intensity exercise with complete dedication is difficult due to practical reasons. We all have to take part in the race of life. Maintaining a healthy balance among work, personal life, leisure and health become difficult for most. Whenever people find themselves at the crossroads where they need to make a compromise, health is the first to go. So, exercise is very easy to take the back seat if you are especially not a die-hard health freak. It is very unlikely as in that case, you wouldn't have been looking for the reasons to lose weight.

Exercise is an excellent way to maintain your good health. Intermittent fasting will give a boost to your fat burning abilities if you exercise. You can multiply the impact of exercise with the help of intermittent fasting.

Intermittent fasting helps in the production of growth hormones. This is a special fat buster hormone and helps in the building of muscle mass. If you exercise in the fasted state, the results can be astonishing. Therefore, you must do regular exercise while you follow intermittent fasting.

Discussing pills and surgery would be of no use here as they are also equally unsustainable ways to losing weight. They have their own perils and cause more problems than benefits.

The best and most sustainable way to lose weight is through intermittent fasting. You can easily lose weight if you follow a healthy lifestyle and have healthy eating habits. Coupling this with regular exercise can give you unimaginable results.

The next few chapters will discuss in detail the ways in which you can follow intermittent fasting.

Chapter 7

INTERMITTENT FASTING METHODS

Intermittent fasting is the way to good health. Each intermittent fasting method has its own benefits. No one method is superior to the other. The type of intermittent fasting that would work best for you would depend on the kind of goal you set.

Intermittent fasting has several benefits apart from weight loss. People follow intermittent fasting for:

- Losing weight and belly fat
- Gaining lean muscle mass
- Improving blood sugar levels
- Improving insulin sensitivity
- Anti-aging effects

There are other similar benefits of intermittent fasting. In order to get the best results, your goal must be clear. That way, you will be able to choose the plan that will work best for you.

Intermittent fasting in its essence will always remain the same. All the methods will also ultimately lead to the same results. However, some methods will lead to one type of results faster than the other. It is similar to working out in the gym. The aim is always the same to lose fat and gain muscles. All types of exercises will help in burning calories. But, high-intensity interval training will lead to better results faster, usually weight training will help you in bulking up muscles. Exercises for specific muscles will help in muscle building in those areas faster. Intermittent methods also work in a similar fashion.

Therefore, to get the best results you must:

- Set clearly defined goals for yourself
- Choose the best intermittent fasting method that severs that purpose
- Adopt a suitable exercise routine and plan your meals accordingly
- Start making slow but consistent changes in your lifestyle and food
- Inform friends and family about your plans so that they can play a supportive role.

A Very Important Thing To Do Is To NOT Rush the Process

Over-enthusiasm is a common phenomenon, and most of the time it causes more damage than good. It happens in everything. You join a gym. The first day when you start the exercise there is no pain or fatigue. You start to do exercise and will feel that the people who have been training for years are only doing small sets. The end result is never good. The next day you only have cramps, pain, and fatigue. You find yourself unable to go to the gym and your plan fails miserably.

This happens with most things. The experienced people who were doing things in moderation weren't wrong. It is not a one-day thing.

If you want your intermittent fasting to be successful:

- ➢ Never rush the process.
- ➢ Never choose a tough plan to begin with
- ➢ Don't be Over-Enthusiastic
- ➢ Always try to adapt yourself to the plan

- Start with easy things and then move on to the next when you get habitual
- Don't do anything to boast
- Give every new step time of a few weeks before moving on to the next step
- Remain consistent and do not take frequent breaks

Don't Set Ambiguous Goals- Set Easily Achievable Goals

The worse thing than not having goals is to have ambiguous goals. Such goals can change easily. You can always play with such goals or rubbish them altogether.

Always set clear goals. Losing weight is not a goal, losing 5 pounds in a month or in a fortnight is. You must be very clear about the expectations you make and if you keep your expectation levels very low, then you may not put any effort into low. If you set them very high, then you may not achieve them and end up feeling disheartened.

The best way is to set an achievable goal for which you can take out the required time and invest effort.

Have small milestones so that you can remain motivated while you reach the ultimate goal.

Develop a Clear Understanding of the Chosen Intermittent Fasting Method

The basic concept of all intermittent fasting methods are the same. It is just a variation of the fasting and feasting windows. However, the plans still have their subtle differences. Before choosing a plan, you must make a conscious decision and do a thorough research about it. Do not invest your time and energy half-heartedly. Study the method properly and understand the things required of you, and the main rules clearly for the best results. You must have the pros and cons of any specific program in mind before diving in.

Don't Get Disheartened by the Small Road Bumps

Like every effort in life, even intermittent fasting may not go smoothly in the beginning. Depending upon your schedule, patience, or level of control on temptation, you may feel defeated at times. This is a normal course of life. We all falter at times. If you ever give in to temptations sometimes, do not get disheartened. Start again with a clean slate. Do not let yourself give in to small surrenders.

Every person has a unique body time and it may react differently. Some people start getting very fast results while others take more time, but this isn't something to worry about. Your body may take some time to show results but it will ultimately show them. You can also face some side-effects at the beginning like a headache, nausea and the feeling of weakness. These are temporary symptoms and there is nothing to worry about as these symptoms will subside soon. Most people face these issues as caffeine withdrawal symptoms. If you have been living of an excessive amount of sugar, then you also may face these symptoms. Your body gets rid of the toxic material and cleans itself. These symptoms are a result of that process itself.

Start with a clear mind and determination and you will be able to achieve all your health goals through intermittent fasting.

Chapter 7 (a)

THE 5:2 FASTS

People consider this to be the easiest plan. In reality, you don't fast on any day while you follow this plan. However, this doesn't reduce the effectiveness of the plan.

This plan has two portions.

I. The 5 normal eating days

On these days you will not be following any fasting plan and therefore, you can eat normally. But, you must use this liberty with great caution. If you keep on eating unhealthy food these days, the results wouldn't be very positive. You will have to follow restraint. You can pick any 5 days of the week as your normal eating days. The 2 fasting days will have to in between these 5 days. You must eat and healthy and balanced diet on these remaining 5 days.

II. The 2 fasting days

The 2 days in this part aren't actually fasting days. However, you will have to follow severe calorie restriction on these 2 days. The calorie allowance for women on these days is 500 calories. For men, the whole calorie allowance is of 600. This means that you will have to adjust all your meals within this calorie range. There is no definite rule for consuming these calories. You can consume all the calories in a single meal and remain in a fasted state for the rest of the day, or divide them into 3 small meals. The decision will be completely yours.

A total of 500-600 calories aren't much and therefore, the trick is to choose the food items that fill you up without adding many calories. Keeping leafy green vegetables is the best bet on these days. The leafy greens have a negligible amount of calories and they fill you up. The digestive fiber in them also helps your gut.

You can also add eggs, grilled chicken, fish, vegetable soup and other such things. You will have to ensure that you do not breach the calorie count.

The fasting days restrict your calorie intake to 25%. However, the bigger problem is not the lower calorie intake.

Your stomach functions in a very time-bound manner. Every day your stomach starts releasing a hunger hormone called 'Ghrelin' at the regular time of your meals. It acts like clockwork. You must have felt that you start feeling hungry every day around the same time. It is the hunger hormone doing the trick. The thing that makes the 5:2 plan a bit difficult to follow is this hormone. You can never get used to this routine as you follow a different routine 5 days a week in no specific order.

This challenge makes this plan so effective and it forces your body to start burning the fat for fulfilling the calorie deficit.

This plan is much better for the people who can't keep regular fasts or who need to eat on a regular basis. Even if they need to eat 3 times a day, this plan would work for them.

The results are a bit slow as it is a beginners plan but it brings your body in order. You can also choose this plan to get accustomed to longer fasts.

Chapter 7 (6)

THE 12 HOUR FASTS

This is the easiest in the series of intermittent fasting where you actually remain in the fasted state. The 5:2 plan should be treated as an exception as you do not observe an actual fast.

The Method

The method of fast is very simple. You will have to remain in the fasted state for at least 12 hours consecutively. This may sound a lot for some but in reality, it is nothing. On an average day, you remain in the fasted state for 7-9 hours without any difficulty. This is a time when you are sleeping. Although you are not consciously keeping the fast, your body still remains in the fasted state and that counts. You simply need to add a couple of more hours before or after you sleep.

The best way to do this is to eat a couple of hours before you go to bed. Eating a few hours before going to bed is a healthy habit anyway. It gives your body the chance to digest the food properly. Hence, you can avoid several digestive issues.

If you don't eat 3 hours before you go to bed, you would feel the need to eat anyway. Normal sleeping hours range from 7-9 hours. You would simply have to avoid eating anything or drinking tea or coffee for 1 or 2 hours. If you feel the urge you can still have unsweetened black tea or coffee. They do not add any calorie to your system and therefore, you will still remain in the fasted state.

The Ways to Make it Work

The best way to succeed with this plan is to first create healthy gaps between your meals. It means that you should begin by limiting yourself to only 3 meals a day. Frequent snacking is a habit that will make your fasting difficult, and leads to cravings for food. You are not really hungry but you feel the need to eat after a short interval. When you eliminate the snacks from your routine, your body adapts to the change. You stop feeling the need to eat for 3-4 hours after your meals.

The Impact

The 12-hour fasts are simple and easy. However, this doesn't undermine the efficiency of the fasts. Studies on mice have shown that even the 12-hours fasts can help you in losing weight. The study had two groups of mice with the test group allowed to eat only 12 hours a day. The other group of mice was also fed the same number of calories but they were allowed to eat as and when they liked. Within a month the test group showed considerable improvement in weight and their vital parameters also improved.

Meal Management

The First Meal

One important thing that can make your fasts convenient is your management of the meals. If you are having 3 meals a day type routine, it is best for you to have your first meal of the day as the biggest meal. The reason is simple. This is the meal that gets the largest amount of time to get digested while you are comparatively more active. You can have a nutritious meal and process it more effectively.

The Second Meal

The second meal or lunch should be lighter. Having a very heavy lunch would make you feel drowsy and make it difficult to work. This part of the meal should have food items that are easy to digest. The gap between the lunch and dinner progressively goes down as you move ahead with intermittent fasting. Your focus should always remain to have breakfast as late as possible so that the need for lunch can be eliminated. When you have a healthy and fulfilling breakfast the need and appetite for lunch goes down automatically. So, you should get into a habit of having a light lunch. Fruits and salads in the lunch work the best.

The Third Meal

The third meal of the day or the dinner should be the lightest. This part of the meal needs to be processed by your body in an inactive state. Your body is busiest normally when you are asleep. Stuffing yourself with food will put you under undue pressure. You should remember to have the smallest meal at dinner and eat food full of digestive fiber is the best thing to have when it comes to dinner time meals.

Most people fear that having a light dinner would make them feel early. They have no reason to worry as this is not how the body works. Your appetite is not controlled by the amount of food you consume but by the time when you consume it. It means that if you have formed a habit of having dinner at 6 pm, and breakfast at 8 am then your body can easily manage to remain in the fasted state in-between. You wouldn't have to put any extra effort to make that work.

Even if you feel the hunger pangs in the initial stage, you can have green tea, black tea, black coffee or fresh lime water. These beverages work very well in dousing your hunger pangs. They make you feel more satisfied. However, the important rule to follow is to avoid using sugar. The main aim of intermittent fasting is to avoid the intake of calories in the fasting state. Addition of calories will activate your digestive system as well as your pancreas. This is one thing you would want to avoid if you want to get weight loss benefits.

For beginners, the 12-hour fasts are the best as they put you in the game. You can get habitual of short fasting periods, and then you can move to the longer fasts.

Chapter 7 (c)

THE 16:8 PLAN- THE LEAN GAIN METHOD

This is one of the most sustainable intermittent fasting plans of all and brings great results. It can be followed in the long-term and gives you great health benefits. It is also called the Leangain fasting method as it helps you in reducing body fat and gaining muscle mass. So, if you are planning to have a chiseled body, then following this fasting routine with a healthy diet and exercise can do the trick for you.

The 16:8 Plan for Men

The 16:8 intermittent fasting requires you have to fast for 16 hours and have an eating window of 8 hours.

The 16:8 Plan for Women

In the case of women, following a fasting window of 14 hours and the eating window of 10 hours gives more beneficial results. This is due to rapid hormonal changes taking place in their body.

The 8-hour eating window is the case of men, and 10-hour eating window is the case of women is the time in when you can eat. There is no calorie restriction in this eating window. You can eat pretty much any amount of food you want, however, stuffing yourself is never advisable.

You must eat only till the point when you start feeling reasonably satisfied. This is because you will start feeling satisfied soon after you have eaten a decent amount of food. The only thing to consider here is that you must eat healthy food in this window. Fill up your meals with a good balance of macronutrients. It should have a healthy mix of carbohydrates, proteins, and fat. Eat whole foods as they have a lot of digestive fiber and slow digesting carbohydrates. It gives you energy and stops unnecessary insulin spikes.

The best thing about the 16:8 intermittent fasting plan is that it can be followed easily in the daily routine. You wouldn't feel awkward while going out with friends as there is no calorie restriction. You are free to eat whatever you like without feeling the guilt.

The 8-10 hours of eating window give you an ample amount of time to eat. You will not feel starved or repressed like in all other diets. This factor alone makes the 16:8 plan more sustainable than other weight loss diets.

The Routine

You can choose the eating window as per your convenience. For instance, if you normally feel very hungry early in the morning then you can start your eating window in the morning. However, if you are more of a night person and start your day a bit late, then you can shift your eating window to the latter part of the day. The only important thing here is to observe a minimum of 14-16 hours of fast as per your gender.

The 16:8 Plan for Morning People

The morning people can begin their eating windows at 9 or 10 in the morning. This is almost the time when you start your working day. You can take a healthy breakfast and start your work. Have your lunch a bit early, and the last meal of the day by 5 or 6 in the evening. Try to shift your breakfast as far into the day as possible.

For all practical purposes, you'll find that after having a healthy breakfast the need to have lunch is negligible.

In case you want to have lunch to be very moderate. If you eat stuff that is heavy, you will not be able to feel hungry by the time of your last meal before the fasting window opens.

The 8-hour window from the perspective of a person who has had a heavy breakfast is very small. Adjusting three big meals into this window can become a problem. You need to keep in mind that if you want to have an early breakfast then having dinner early in the day is the best option for you.

Having an early dinner also gives you other health benefits. When you have your dinner around 5 or 6, your body gets a good 4-5 hours to digest the food before you go to sleep.

The 16:8 Plan for the Night owls

The people who are more of night owls also don't need to worry at all. Intermittent fasting remains the same for them. If you work till late at night and start your day in the later part of the morning, then there is nothing to worry about. You simply need to shift the first meal of your day a bit further.

For instance, you take the first meal of your day around 12. You get an eating window up to 8 at night. You simply need to ensure that you do not go to sleep immediately after taking your dinner which you wouldn't do anyway. This will give you enough time to digest your food. All the benefits would remain the same in that case.

It's Simple

Following a 16:8 intermittent fasting routine is very simple. Your intermittent fasting days remain the same as all other days. You do not need to make special preparations or take out extra time from your schedule.

The biggest reason for most of the weight loss measures is that they require a lot of effort, time, and money. Whenever you are not able to give either of them, the efforts start failing. In the case of intermittent fasting, neither of them is required.

If you are following a good eating regimen, then the results will get amplified. However, you will still be getting the benefits of intermittent fasting even if you fail to get healthy meals.

The same is the case with exercise. If you are able to work out on an empty stomach, your fat burning would get amplified. Your body is able to produce several hormones like the growth hormone and the adrenaline that help in fat burning. These hormones can only be produced when your body is the in fasting state. When you have a high concentration of these hormones, the results of exercise are much better. You will burn the fat faster and gain muscles. But, in case, you are not able to workout due to one reason or the other, you'll still be able to lose weight and remain healthy.

Following an intermittent fasting, the routine has no extra cost. In fact, your food expenses and your medical bills would go down with time.

You will be able to enjoy better health, higher brain function, better digestive system, and immunity. Your liver function would improve, the cholesterol issues would go down, and you will lose a lot of belly fat.

Some Important Tips for Following 16:8 Intermittent Fasting Plan are:

You must drink plenty of water. Remaining hydrated is important. Your body goes through a detoxification process on intermittent fasting. Water helps in flushing these toxins out of your body.

Drinking a lot of water keeps you full without adding any calories. You will be easily able to manage hunger pangs with water.

As your body undergoes the detoxification process, you can experience mild headaches or lightheadedness. There is no need to worry from these symptoms as they will vanish once your body detoxifies. Unsweetened black tea or coffee will help you in these symptoms. However, you must limit your intake of tea or coffee to one or two cups only.

Have healthy meals with a lot of protein. A Protein-rich diet keeps you feeling fuller for much longer.

The first meal of the day should be the largest meal of the day. This gives your body ample amount of time to process the food. You must start lowering the quantity of food you eat in the subsequent meals.

These simple tips can help you a lot in remaining healthy and losing a lot of belly fat easily.

Chapter 7 (d)

THE 20:4 INTERMITTENT PLAN- THE WARRIOR FASTS

As the name suggests, this intermittent fasting plan involves fasting for 20 hours in a day and permits only four hours of eating window. The longer fasting window gives your body more time to digest the food and puts pressure on it to burn more fat to produce energy.

You can have better fat loss results through this plan. However, fat loss is not the only benefit of this intermittent fasting plan. It is among the most favorite fasting plans of bodybuilders all over the globe. The reason is very simple. It leads to fat loss and development of lean muscle mass. It means that you'll not only be able to lose a lot of fat through this plan but it will also help you in bulking up.

If you are wondering that fasting may reduce the stamina to do hard weight training, then your worries are misplaced. Nature has a plan for everything. Your body stores energy in two separate forms. When you eat anything, the first part of the energy is instantly used up by your cells directly with the help of insulin. Then the second part of surplus energy gets stored in the liver and muscles as glycogen. These muscle glycogen stores have a unique property. They can only be used by the muscles as where they are stored. When you exercise in the fasted state, these glycogen stores get used for the work out of specific muscles and hence, there is no problem of stamina. The remaining third part of excess energy gets stored as fat in your body. This can be used to supply energy to your body in case there is any shortage of energy. So, even in a fasted state, you can do exercise without any problem. Several studies in athletes have shown that high-intensity exercises in a fasted state have minimum impact on their performance.

This is one of the most natural fasting plans for us. Since the very beginning, procurement of food had been a struggle for mankind. Our ancestors struggled for hours and days in the end to get food. They also lacked the resources to store food. So, the natural way was to hunt or gather whatever they could and eat it in one go. This gave them enough energy to survive until the next hunt.

This is a reason our body finds this routine to be very natural and responds to it very well.

The 4-hour eating window in the 20:4 plan is all that you have to eat. You can eat whatever you want. The food should be nutritious as you will need to consume the daily requirement of protein and fat in one go. Here, you must remember that protein and fat-rich diet is heavy and hence, initially eating a lot of it is very difficult. You will develop the ability to eat your fill in one go at a slow pace.

Longer fasting hours ensure that your insulin sensitivity improves. It also helps in fighting with any kind of chronic inflammation in your body. Your liver and pancreas get a great relief and your overall health improves tremendously.

High-intensity exercise and a nutritious meal are the two main requirements for the success of this routine. However, as a word of caution, you must not begin with 20:4 routine in the first place.

It is a tough routine, and acclimatizing your body to the tough fasting routine is very important.

Therefore, you should start with a 16:8 plan and then move on to the 20:4 routine slowly.

You Must Keep in Mind the Following Things Before Taking Up 20:4 Intermittent Fasting

- ➢ Increase your appetite as you will only get one meal in a day to consume all the nutrition. It becomes a problem for many first-timers.
- ➢ You should develop a busy schedule, as fighting the hunger pangs can get difficult initially.
- ➢ Start by pushing your morning meal towards the end of the day. The biggest problem people face on this routine is to fight with the morning hunger pangs.
- ➢ You must stay away from foods that lead to craving. Frequent snacking and munching habits can pose a real problem for you.

Some Key Notes for the Success of 20:4 Intermittent Fasting

- Go slow but remain consistent. Never take up 20:4 fasting as a challenge.
- It is undoubtedly a tough regimen. You will have to do high-intensity workouts on a single diet. It won't be the hunger that would hurt the most but the craving to eat like others. The best way to deal with the problem is to make your way up the road slowly.
- Start by a shorter fasting routine and then start shifting your meals further. From 3 meals a day to 2, and then merging it with the last meal of the day is the best way to do it. A slow transition is a key to 20:4 fasting success.
- You must always remain positive and resolute. This is not a routine for the faint hearted ones.
- This is also not a routine for the part-timers. You cannot have cheat days. A single cheat day will mean that your cravings will get stronger, and you will want to take more cheat days.

- The better, healthier, and nutritious food you'll eat, the easier it will be to fight cravings and work out hard.
- Never be apprehensive of your success. If you are determined to make it a success, it will be so.
- Drink more and more electrolytes. Your body will go through heavy detoxification in this process. It will make you healthier and energetic. However, you will lose a lot of water and minerals in the process. Keep supplementing them through electrolytes. Adding sea salt to your water along with minerals like potassium and magnesium is always the best.
- This routine can change you from within. You will not only get a better physique but your mental clarity and focus will also increase. You will have better control over your decisions and it requires overcoming many mental hurdles.

You should go for it if you want to have a good physique.

Chapter 7 (e)

EAT-STOP-EAT PLAN

This fasting routine was designed by Brad Pilon. It raises the bar to a higher level. In this routine, you need to fast for 24 hours once or twice a week.

It is tougher as your body will never get used to this regimen. It is a bit taxing to your body, however, the results are incredible.

Eat-Stop-Eat intermittent fasting routine has several health benefits and quick weight loss is one among them. You can lose a lot of weight very quickly through this routine. It also helps in detoxifying your body.

Your body goes through a detoxification process as the fasting duration is quite long. It develops a positive stress response which is very good for your body.

This fasting routine is not new. It is practiced in several religions as a ritual. People follow it and get great health benefits. The only important thing to remember in this fast is that you cannot overeat on the eating days. You will have to keep your food intake normal. Keeping yourself well hydrated is also important as your body will be undergoing detoxification.

It is one of the most researched fasting methods all over the world, and the results have been incredible. Studies have shown that people can lose up to 4% of their fat mass over a period of 21 days. This means fat mass can be as high as 2.5% in this short span. This fasting protocol is also very helpful in increasing the insulin sensitivity in the body. Most of the animal studies conducted through this method have demonstrated that the stress response of the control group improved considerably.

The results of the fast can vary according to the age, gender, and amount of exercise done by the practitioner, but the overall results have been very promising.

There is no doubt in the fact that it is a difficult routine to follow as the body can get off balance. Observing a complete day of fast and then having a complete eating day can become taxing. But, looking at the results, this routine is quite popular in people trying to lose weight quickly.

Key Tips for Eat-Stop-Eat Intermittent Fasting

- You must drink plenty of water. Your body will be doing a lot of detoxification. Not drinking enough water can lead to the development of stones.
- Drink unsweetened fresh lime water on the fasting days as it will help in detoxification. It will flush out all the toxic material from your body and prevent the buildup of stones.
- Your eating days should have a lot of protein in the meals. It will help you in remaining satiated for long and also prevent loss of muscle mass.
- Overeating of non-fast days can be a bad idea. However, you do not need to follow calorie restriction. Simply eat nutritious food with lots of fiber, protein, and fat to keep you going strong.
- Watching others eat while you are fasting can be tough as you will have to exercise great self-control. The easy way to avoid such

situations is to keep your friends and family in the loop. This way you can easily prevent the temptation of food when others are not eating in your sight.

The Eat-Stop-Eat routine in itself is very simple. You simply need to avoid calorie intake on the fasting days and eat normally on the eating days. Besides avoiding binge eating, there is no other precaution that you need to take.

You can begin your fasts as per your convenience. It is best to begin the fasts in the morning as the toughest time is the last part of the fast. In this case, it will be the time when you are sleeping and hence, most inconveniences can be avoided.

However, this is not a compulsion. If you feel it fit, you can begin your fasts in the evenings too.

The timing of the fast has no impact on your fat loss or other health benefits.

Chapter 7 (f)

ALTERNATE DAY FASTS

Alternate day fasts are an extension of the 5:2 plan. Here, in place of having two days of calorie restriction, you follow it every other day.

Alternate day fasting requires you to have only 25% of your calorie intake on the fasting days. This means that the options to eat on the fasting days get limited. You will have to focus on getting all your calories from fats, lean proteins, and vegetables.

This is a very good way to lose weight for those people who have erratic food habits. It helps you in controlling your food intake. There are no complete fasting days and therefore even the people with diabetes or blood sugar issues can also keep these fasts on the advice of their doctor.

The trick to succeed with this plan is to completely avoid the intake of food items having refined sugar and starchy foods.

When you begin any kind of fasting protocol, becoming conscious of the kind of food you eat is important. You must develop a habit of reading the labels. Most processed food items have refined sugar in them. Food products with sugar, syrups, fructose must be avoided. Such items add empty calories to your system without bringing any digestive fiber. They raise your insulin levels and cause a number of problems. You should avoid them as best as possible.

The Positive Effects of Alternate Days Fasts:

- ➢ Accelerated weight loss
- ➢ Help in lowering the risk of Type 2 Diabetes
- ➢ Better for your heart health
- ➢ Helps in managing your blood pressure

These are only some of the benefits of alternate day fasting. The best thing fasting does to you is it helps your body in processing food. Your body gets the time to manage lots of processes that become overworked due to constant abuse of frequent meals.

Food is an important requirement of our body. However, you must always remember that it is simply a fuel. Overfilling the tank leads to wastage.

It can cause a number of problems. It is like overcharging a battery. If you keep your phone always on charging, the battery power would weaken. Eating sensibly is always the best option.

Improving your eating habits is also very important. The more responsible you become, the better your health will be. One important thing to remember on any kind of fasting is that you must never get off a fast with heavy heating. This will make you feel bloated. You should break your fast with something light. Give your body some time to process that food and then have a proper meal. Never force your body to fast for long and then process large quantities of food. It will get confused and wouldn't be able to work properly.

Chapter 8

The Science Behind Intermittent Fasting

Intermittent fasting works wonders for our body. It is a practice which brings your body in its natural routine.

- ➤ It helps your body to get an ample amount of time to digest food.
- ➤ Short eating windows ensure that your calorie intake remains responsible
- ➤ It helps your body in burning fat

Fat has become a dangerous word in the current age. There is a hysteria that fat is bad and unhealthy. However, most of these claims have no basis. Excess of fat is bad. For that matter, an excess of anything is bad.

Consider the simple fact that oxygen is vital for our lives. We can't breathe without oxygen. But, the percentage of oxygen in the air we breathe is not absolute. In fact, it is not even the major constituent. If someone is forced to inhale pure oxygen, the results would be very bad and prolonged exposure will lead to lung failure and death.

Likewise, fat is important for our body. It is the excess of fat that causes the problem. Our body has some very important roles for fat.

Why Do We Accumulate Fat?

We have been through millions of years of evolutionary process. Our bodies have been hardwired to survive in all conditions. We have survived the stone age when our ancestors lived as nomads. They didn't have any steady source of food. At times they got food in abundance and at others, they didn't. Our bodies have got adapted to those settings. Our ancestors have also been through the ice ages, droughts and famines.

All these times have taught our bodies to survive in any condition. The fat in our body is also a part of this survival mechanism. During the periods of feasts, our body keeps accumulating fat. It protects the fat deposits fiercely as they prove crucial to survival in the times of fast.

This is the prime reason for the difficult fat burning process. Your body will never start burning fat till there is a ready supply of energy. When our ready supply of energy gets depleted, our body can survive on this fat for days and even months. This explains the attachment of our bodies towards fat.

However, the problem is that the times of food uncertainty are long gone. Now, you can easily get food even in times of floods, famines, and droughts. But, your body has still not come out of that mode. This makes the accumulation of fat easy and shedding of fat a challenge.

How Intermittent Fasting Helps in Fat Burning?

It creates an artificial demand for energy. Intermittent fasting creates a temporary shortage of energy. You need to stop consuming food for a definite number of hours a day. But, your body doesn't stop working in this period. It keeps burning fuel. The energy from food consumed by you is short lived. It can only last from 8-12 hours. If you fast for longer than this, your body will have no other option than to burn the energy deposits. This leads to the effect of fat burning.

Advantages of Burning Fat

- ➢ Burning fat has several advantages besides the obvious weight loss benefit.
- ➢ You can stay away from several health disorders
- ➢ You can prevent lifestyle disorders like diabetes and hypertension
- ➢ The risk of heart diseases also are lower as your body starts using the cholesterol and triglycerides
- ➢ Your risk of chronic inflammation also goes down
- ➢ You will feel more lively and energetic

How Does It Happen?

Like burning carbohydrate, your body also has a process for burning fat. The process of burning body fat is called ketosis. In this process, your body starts utilizing fat and converts it into ketones which your body derives energy from.

Ketones provide you a high amount of energy and they are a clean fuel source. All the myths concerning the ketones have no ground. People with diabetes have high ketone levels and may go through ketoacidosis but that is an entirely different thing. High insulin levels are responsible for the problem and not fat burning.

Some Important Facts About Ketones are:

- Your body loves to run on ketones.
- When your body is going through ketosis, it can burn fat faster and your health biomarkers improve considerably.
- You feel less fatigue. Your cognitive function improves considerably.
- You feel less stress and anxiety.
- You will have better focus and memory.
- You will face fewer problems with high blood pressure.
- You will gain more muscle mass.
- Intermittent fasting helps you in taking your body to that stage.

Intermittent Fasting and Ketosis

Intermittent fasting involves observing longer fasting windows. Ideally, 16 hours of fasting for men and 14 hours of fasting for women should be the beginning of an intermittent fasting routine. After 8-12 hours of fasting, the insulin levels in your blood go down. This facilitates the production of growth hormones and adrenaline hormones which helps a lot with fat burning. When you get accustomed to this routine, you can easily increase your fasting periods and enjoy good health.

Once the process starts, you will experience faster fat burning and muscle mass buildup. It is the preferred routine of bodybuilders all around the globe. The longer your fasting period, the better your fat burning would get.

Intermittent fasting is a reliable method of fat loss. It is also a process that ensures overall good health. So, in case you are simply looking for good health and improved quality of life, then intermittent fasting is deffinetly an ideal routine for you.

Intermittent fasting doesn't require you to go an extra mile for good health. You can simply begin by limiting the number of hours in which you eat. The longer you would go without eating, the better your digestion and other functions would get. You will also be free to eat as much as you want. There is no calorie restriction in place. In fact, a rich diet filled with all the macro and micro-nutrients will help you in improving your health.

Chapter 9

Fat Burning Element of Intermittent Fasting

Intermittent fasting simplifies many things for your body. It gives your body the time to digest food properly and bring harmony among various organ functions. However, before you understand the functioning of intermittent fasting, it is important to understand the cause of most of the problems in your body.

If there is one thing that causes most of the problems in your body, then it is undoubtedly insulin resistance. Insulin is one of the most important hormones in your body. It is an agent that helps in energy absorption.

Functions of Insulin

Whenever you eat something, the food gets converted into glucose, which then mixes into your bloodstream and increases your blood glucose levels. However, your cells cannot accept this glucose directly. This is where insulin comes into play. Your pancreas senses the increased blood glucose levels and releases an insulin hormone. This hormone binds to your cells and enables them to absorb glucose to get energy. The mitochondria in the cells then use this glucose to convert it into energy.

Problems with Poor Reception of Insulin

Your body needs to be very sensitive to this insulin hormone. If there is even a little resistance to this insulin hormone, then your cells will not be able to accept glucose. Your blood glucose levels will increase drastically and it can be fatal. This is the stage which leads to diabetes and it must be avoided at all costs.

The problem begins when your body stops responding to insulin hormone in a normal way. This can occur due to a number of reasons but the biggest reason is high exposure to insulin. High exposure to insulin occurs when you keep eating at frequent intervals.

The Process of Insulin Production

Whenever you eat, your pancreas release insulin. Any meal takes around 8-12 hours to get digested completely. This means that after any meal, the insulin is present for 8-12 hours in your blood. If you keep eating at regular intervals, the pancreas has to pump more and more insulin, which can create insulin resistance. This is bad as you as cells stop responding or respond slowly to insulin.

It means that your blood sugar levels remain high and your pancreas has to pump more and more insulin to stabilize the blood sugar levels. Your pancreas becomes overworked and the insulin concentration in your body increases.

High Insulin Leads to Fat Accumulation

Insulin is a major hormone. It has several functions other than binding with the cells for storing glucose. It is also the fat storage hormone. When the glucose levels are high and your cells cannot accept any more glucose, insulin starts storing glucose in the liver and muscles as glycogen. However, glycogen stores are small and then it triggers the fat hormones to store the access energy as fat. So, higher insulin levels will lead to greater fat accumulation. This is one of the reasons that people with high food intake become fat. Their body is usually in the reception mode and keeps storing energy as fat.

Problems in Fat Burning

Till there is insulin in your bloodstream, any kind of fat burning will not take place. The reason is very simple, your body is constantly getting signals to store fat. The insulin levels will remain high if you keep eating at regular intervals as every meal will lead to an insulin release. Which overall becomes a vicious cycle.

This is How Intermittent Fasting Helps

Intermittent fasting helps you in breaking this vicious cycle. In intermittent fasting, you will have to observe a minimum fasting period of 14-16 hours. This can be extended to 48 hours as per your convenience. We have learned that the presence of insulin is for 8-12 hours after your last meal. This means that your body will observe periods when there is a complete absence of insulin in your blood. It is the single best thing for your health in general and fat burning, in particular.

When you go without food for more than 8 hours, insulin levels go down. Your pancreas does not get any signal to pump any more insulin as there is no blood glucose release. This absence of insulin helps in creating insulin sensitivity. Your cells start responding better to insulin. This is good for you in more ways than one. Firstly, the load on your pancreas goes down. The pancreas does not remain overworked anymore. This improves the function of the pancreas. Secondly, the amount of insulin needed to process glucose also decreases with better insulin sensitivity. It means that the amount of insulin present in your blood at any given point will not be excessive. It is a great improvement in your health, and other hormones that get inhibited due to the presence of insulin can respond better.

As we discussed earlier, insulin is the major fat storage hormone. Till there is the presence of insulin in your blood, your body will not start burning fat as it is in fat storage mode. Once your insulin levels go down, your body will start using energy deposits in the body for functioning. Your body can only produce most of the fat burning hormones like the Growth Hormone and adrenaline only when there is no insulin in your blood. The absence of insulin triggers the production of these hormones which, in turn, lead to fat loss.

One of the biggest benefits of intermittent fasting is creating insulin sensitivity. It not only helps you in burning fat faster but keeps you away from the dangers of problems like Type 2 Diabetes, obesity, heart problems, and hypertension.

Problems with Diets and Other Weight Loss Measures

You must remember that lowering the calorie intake is not going to help you with weight loss. People who lose weight on diets and other strict calorie restriction plans are generally losing the water weight. This is very easy for it to come back and you do not lose fat at all. Apart from that, these weight loss methods are not sustainable. There is a time limit for any diet, and you cannot remain on a diet forever. Whenever you get off the diet, same problems will recur. The same goes for high-intensity exercises and workouts.

Fat burning is a completely different process. Your body is generally running on a carbohydrate fuel. The food you eat has a very high percentage of carbohydrates. It gets converted into glucose and your body loves to burn it as it is easy to burn and gives instant energy. Fat burning requires complete switching of the energy mode. Your body will need to switch from burning carbohydrates to burning fat. This cannot be done if you are eating frequently and getting a regular supply of carbohydrates through your meals.

Intermittent fasting along with the right food can lead to fat burning. It simply forces your body to look for other energy sources rather than easy carbohydrate fuel. It improves the insulin levels in your body and triggers fat burning. The weight lost through intermittent fasting is an actual fat loss.

> If you want to lose fat and reduce your belly size, then intermittent fasting is the right way to do so.

- If you want to regulate the insulin levels in your blood, then intermittent fasting is the solution for you.
- If you want to avoid the dangers of heart problems, then intermittent fasting is the best method for it.
- Intermittent fasting reduces your blood glucose levels. It helps in fat burning and triggers fat burning hormones.
- It helps in reducing cholesterol, LDL, and triglycerides in your blood leading to a healthy heart.

It is very easy to implement and a long-lasting measure. You only need to do one thing and that is limiting the number of hours in which you consume food and observe longer fasting hours. Only this step will solve most of the problems for you.

Chapter 10

HEALTH BENEFITS OF INTERMITTENT FASTING

Intermittent fasting is simply not a weight loss measure. It helps in overall improvement of your health. Your body will feel better and respond better. You will be able to stay healthy and fit.

There are several health issues in which intermittent fasting has shown commendable results. If you are also facing these issues you can consult your physician and try the intermittent fasting for help.

Improving Heart Health

Health is one of the most important and sensitive organs. If obesity has the highest impact on one organ then it is the heart. The cholesterol levels go high, the blood pressure increases and they ultimately affect the functioning of the heart. Heart diseases are the leading cause of preventable deaths in the US. They also cost a lot in treatment.

Heart diseases are complex as the impact of malfunctioning of other processes is also high on the heart. Intermittent fasting helps you in easing the pressure on your body. It starts healing your body in a systematic way.

- ➢ Your insulin levels improve. Improved insulin levels help you in managing fat better.
- ➢ Your blood pressure also becomes manageable. It is one of the major causes of heart issues. High blood pressure can put a lot of strain on the heart. Once it comes in control, your heart starts beating easy.
- ➢ Your LDL (Bad Cholesterol) levels go down with intermittent fasting. This cholesterol is responsible for blocking your arteries. It is a major troublemaker. The lower the levels of LDL in your blood, the more you minimize the risks.
- ➢ Your HDL (Good Cholesterol) levels increase. HDL plays an important role in maintaining good heart health and also plays other beneficial roles.

Therefore, if heart health is your concern, intermittent fasting is one of the best ways to suppress your worries.

Lower Risk of Diabetes

Prediabetes and diabetes have emerged as the real dangers in the current times. Poor lifestyle and bad eating habits put you at great risk of diabetes. The 2015 CDC reports state that more than 100 million Americans are fighting with diabetes or prediabetes. The struggle with diabetes is an endless and hopeless battle. There is very little that one can do if in the grip of diabetes. It makes life difficult and you end up needing to compromise on several aspects of life.

However, intermittent fasting can help in battling diabetes. It can also help in to prevent the conversion of prediabetes into diabetes. As you know diabetes is a problem caused by the poor response of your body to insulin. Intermittent fasting is known to help your body by developing insulin sensitivity. Your insulin response improves and you will be able to manage healthy blood sugar levels.

It is a long process and would require you to be patient and consistent, but it is possible. People all over the world are adopting intermittent fasting for preventing or managing diabetes.

Modern medicine has no cure for diabetes. It only focuses on managing diabetes by giving insulin. This is not the solution to the problem. This method of treatment is costly and tiresome too. You can try intermittent fasting along with your medication to get better results. Medical studies have proven that people on intermittent fasting have better blood sugar levels and insulin sensitivity.

Lowers the Risk of Chronic Inflammation

Chronic inflammations are the cause of most serious issues in your body. They keep on causing the damage silently and the problems only emerge when they have blown out of proportion. Liver, kidney, heart, lung, and digestive tract issues are a result of chronic inflammation.

An unhealthy lifestyle and poor food choices are the biggest reasons for chronic inflammation. Obese or overweight people are especially in the risk zone of inflammation. Chronic inflammation is simply your body's overreaction to infections. When your immune system goes in an overdrive it leads to chronic inflammation.

The risk of chronic inflammation will increase if you are:

- Obese or overweight
- Have unhealthy food and poor eating habits
- Live a sedentary lifestyle
- Have a lot of stress

Chronic inflammation not only impairs the functioning of your vital organs it also affects the functioning of your brain. The oxidative stress in your body increases and it stops performing optimally.

Intermittent fasting has a very positive impact on oxidative stress. Oxidative stress is caused due to the imbalance of free radicals in the blood and lack of antioxidants. Intermittent fasting inhibits the production of free radicals and reduces oxidative stress.

Inflammation is not a bad thing in itself, and is just your body's natural response to dealing with problems. However, prolonged inflammation can prove to be dangerous and it should be avoided. Intermittent fasting can help you in fighting inflammation and reversing its adverse effects.

Chapter 11

THINGS TO CHECK BEFORE YOU BEGIN INTERMITTENT FASTING

Intermittent fasting is one of the best ways to maintain good health. It also helps you in burning fat and losing weight. However, it still might not be for you.

You must keep in mind that intermittent fasting is a lifestyle change. It would require you to mend your ways. If you are suffering from some kind of medical condition, a sudden change in lifestyle may affect you adversely.

Taking up any such routine without preparation and knowledge can be risky. You must consider consulting your physician before beginning intermittent fasting if you are taking any medication. This not only lowers the risk of complications but also helps the doctor in taking preventive measures.

If you are healthy and not facing any kind of medical condition, then intermittent fasting is a safe practice. However, there are certain conditions in which you must consult your doctor before beginning intermittent fasting.

History of Eating Disorders

A history of eating disorders should be taken seriously. Intermittent fasting will bring a change into your eating patterns. If in the past you have suffered from any kind of eating disorder, you must consult your physician before beginning intermittent fasting.

Diabetes

If you are suffering from diabetes, prediabetes or have high or low blood sugar level issues, then you must not begin intermittent fasting without consulting your doctor. Intermittent fasting definitely has a positive impact on these conditions but it needs to be monitored. Diabetes can cause your blood sugar levels to fluctuate rapidly. This can put you at risk. Consulting the doctor prior to beginning intermittent fast can help you in doing better. The doctor can help you in regular monitoring and dose adjustment of your medications and insulin.

You must not ignore this step if you are suffering from any of these conditions. regular monitoring of blood sugar level is very important as at times, prolonged fasts can lead to low blood sugar levels. Low blood sugar levels can also be as fatal as high blood sugar. If you ever feel symptoms like fatigue, shakiness or heart palpitation, you must check your blood sugar and consult the doctor immediately.

Under Medication

If you are taking any kind of medication or undergoing a treatment, then you must consult your doctor. Intermittent fasting can interfere in your medication routine or also affect your nutrient intake. It can make the process of healing difficult. You must consult your doctor in such a condition.

Lactating or Pregnant Women

The women in the process of bearing a child or nursing them must stay away from intermittent fasting. Their energy requirements are very high and they also have the added responsibility of feeding another life. Intermittent fasting can cause a problem in this process. It can make them energy deficient.

Some women also face problems in their menstrual cycles and other health concerns while following intermittent fasting. They must consult their physician immediately for medical advice.

People Suffering from Gallbladder Issues

If you have been suffering from gallbladder issues or have gallstones or similar problems, you must avoid intermittent fasting. These problems can become severe with intermittent fasting. You must consult your physician before taking up the fasts.

People with Unregulated Thyroid

Thyroid hormone can go in overdrive while you are on fasts. The management of this metabolic hormone is very important for good health. If you have been facing thyroid issues, then you must consult your physician immediately.

Children and Teenagers

The energy demands of kids and teenagers are very high. They need a lot of nutrients to grow properly. Intermittent fasting can affect their growth. Healthy kids should avoid intermittent fasting in this period. If the kid is suffering from obesity then proper consultation of the physician is strongly advised before beginning the fasts.

Chapter 12

Tips to Succeed with Your Intermittent Fasting Routine

Intermittent fasting is a process and like all processes, you will have your highs and lows. It is very important for you to stay motivated and keep working. You must never allow yourself to feel defeated.

Small hiccups and breaches would happen. There would be times when you would have to attend late night parties. There will be times when you cave into temptation. However, such things shouldn't stop you from getting on your schedule the next day and you should not make it a habit to cheat.

You must remember that the next day of your cheat day will be difficult. Your body would start demanding food at the time of your last day's meals.

To prevent such struggles, it is always best to stick to a schedule.

There are a few things that will not only make your journey easy but will also help you in getting better results.

Walks are Good

Physical activity is a crucial part of burning fat. However, engaging in intense physical activity can become difficult for people struggling with excessive weight. Brisk walks are a completely different story even for such people. You should go for walks every day. This is one activity that will help you in taking away your mind from other things and also give you immense health benefits. Long walks help in burning fat too. You should take walks in the morning or any other time that suits you. Missing the walks is like missing a golden opportunity.

Don't Overstrain Yourself on the Fasting Days

In the beginning, fasting can be a bit taxing. Putting your body under too much strain can become a problem, and can make you start to feel frustrated or agitated. You must take it easy on the fasting days in the beginning. As you get habitual of the fasts, your body will adapt and you can follow your normal routine. If you feel lightheadedness or fatigue then give yourself some rest.

Keep Yourself Occupied

When you are idle, the brain thinks more about food. This is very normal. The best way to avoid the hunger pangs is to keep yourself occupied with things. The more you remain busy, the less you'll think about food.

Don't Indulge in Emotional Eating

Emotional eating is one of the biggest sources of hoarding calories. People start finding pleasure in eating sweets and chocolates as it gives them a dopamine kick. However, it is an unhealthy habit as these things lead to cravings. You will find it difficult to stop at one and will feel the urge to eat a bit more after a short duration. The best way to deal with this problem is to abstain from any kind of emotional eating and maintain your regular eating routine.

Include Healthy Things in Your Diet

A balanced amount of fat and protein in your diet will help you in feeling satisfied. It will prevent any kind of craving. The junk food or unhealthy food only fill you with empty calories, refined sugar, and additives. You must try to stay away from them.

Drink Non-caloric Beverages to Avoid Hunger Pangs

If you feel hungry, having unsweetened beverages like green tea, black tea, black coffee or fresh lime without sugar is the best way to keep hunger pangs at bay. You must avoid sodas.

Do not Give in to the Pressure of the Breakfast

People around you may pressurize you for having breakfast. It has been fed into the brains by the constant display of commercials that breakfast is the healthiest meal of the day. This is just a myth. Your first meal is the healthiest but it doesn't need to be early in the morning. You must follow your fasting window, and have a healthy meal to break your fast whenever your eating window permits you.

Choose a Diet That Works the Best for You

Sticking to a wrong diet can make your journey difficult. You may feel constrained and find it difficult to maintain a healthy routine. Find the items that are healthy and bring them into your diet. Do not go by the trend. If you feel that eating broccoli three times a day is not for you then do not force yourself. Include other items that have a good nutrient base. Include a healthy mix of fat, protein, and fiber in your diet.

Remain Positive

Negativity leads to stress. It is one of the biggest reasons for failure. You must have a positive outlook. Do not go by short-term gains. Intermittent fasting will bring long-term positive changes in your life, so set realistic goals and follow them with conviction.

Chapter 13

Foods That Help and the Foods to Avoid

Intermittent fasting doesn't dictate you much on the things you can eat and the ones you can't. However, this doesn't mean that certain food items will not have a positive or negative impact. You can always accelerate your progress by including a few things and excluding others from your diet.

Few Important Things to Include are:

Water

Water is the most essential thing in intermittent fasting. You will need to drink water and keep yourself hydrated. Your body goes through a lot of detoxification while on intermittent fasting. Not drinking enough water can pose a problem, as water helps in clearing out the toxins from your body which keep you healthy. However, there is one caution that you must take. When you drink more water and your body flushes out toxins, it also flushes out a lot of minerals. This can cause a mineral deficiency. The easy way to counter this problem is to drink water with fresh lime and a pinch of sea salt. This replenishes the minerals and keeps you feeling fresh. Lime also prevents the formation of kidney stones. You should consume at least one lime a day in drinks to prevent the formation of stones.

Fish

Fish is the healthiest source of Omega-3 fatty acids which are antioxidants. They help in reducing oxidative stress and inflammation in your body. Fish has lean meat and very healthy balance of fat and protein. You can eat fish for staying in your calorie range and treating your taste buds too. At least 6 to 8 ounces of fish every day will help you in staying fit and healthy.

Avocado

Avocado is a fat-rich fruit, yet it is very healthy for your body. It provides you the required fat you need in a healthy form. Intermittent fasting can also take a toll on your energy supply, but this tasty fruit can help you in keeping your energy stock full. It is full of monounsaturated fats that are not unhealthy or bad. It is a versatile fruit and can be eaten in any meal you want. Use it in salads, recipes, or eat it as it is, the choice is yours.

Leafy Greens

Leafy greens are very important. They provide you with essential vitamins, minerals, fiber, without adding many calories to your system. You can eat leafy greens in copious amounts if you like. They will have no impact on your calorie intake. leafy greens help in making you feel satisfied for longer. They also help in fighting inflammations and reduce the oxidative stress on your body. You can remain disease free by eating leafy greens regularly. You must eat at least 7-8 cups of leafy greens every day. Things like Kale, broccoli, and lettuce are just some of the healthy leafy greens that you must include in your diet.

Potatoes

Potato is an odd choice when it comes to any weight loss measure. It is starchy and full of calories. Yet, it has made its way into the list for one simple reason, you do need calories too. Boiled or baked potatoes can make full pretty fast and keep you satisfied. Even their skin contains a lot of nutrients. The only thing to keep in mind is that you simply can't fry them.

Eggs

Eggs are great when it comes to having the perfect blend of fat and protein. They are rich in both. Boiled eggs can make you feel satisfied for long. You can have boiled eggs in the morning and easily move to lunchtime without feeling the urge to eat. They also help you in building muscles and provide you with a lot of energy.

Whole Grains

Whole grains are a rich source of dietary fiber and nutrients apart from carbohydrates. Completely avoiding whole grains is not a healthy option. You need the trace minerals obtained from the whole grains to stay healthy. You must include them in your diet. The dietary fiber in whole grains takes a lot of time to get digested. It helps your digestion process and releases energy very slowly. This keeps your digestive system engaged and problems like constipation also ease away.

Probiotics

Probiotics are very important for good health. They have a very positive impact on your gut health. It is hard to believe but your gut has more neurons than your brain. Anything bad that we eat puts a great load on the gut. Even the antibiotics have a very negative impact on gut health. The healthy bacteria living in your gut gets affected by a number of such things. It is essential to also consume probiotic foods like kombucha and kefir.

Legumes

Legumes are a rich source of protein. Including legumes in your diet can help you in feeling full for long. They fill you up and you don't feel the cravings for food. They are easy to digest and do not put extra pressure on your system that other sources of protein like meat exert. They also have a lot of dietary fiber that also helps in improving your digestion process.

Nuts

Nuts are healthy fats. You need fat in your daily diet. Nuts provide you the required fats, antioxidants and minerals in ample quantities. They also make you feel satisfied even if you consume them in small quantities. Nuts like walnuts and almonds have a lot of polyunsaturated fat that is beneficial for you.

The Foods to Avoid

Processed Foods

You must avoid processed food as much as you can. Processed foods have a lot of added sugar. Consuming them in large quantities can damage your weight loss efforts. Processed foods contain a lot of ingredients like MSG to add taste. To increase the shelf life of processed food items, food processing companies use hydrogenated oils, trans fats and other such things in preparing them. This makes the food simply unhealthy for consumption. You must make it a habit to read the label of your food items, and do not purchase things that have sugar, syrup, fructose in the top order of its ingredients. Such foods are full of sugar and will increase obesity. They also cause an insulin spike and you will not be able to control your blood sugar levels.

Low-fat food items are also not healthy. Food marketing companies play with the psyche of the buyers by advertising the food as fat-free. If they take out the fat content from the food it will become tasteless and bland, but they usually add refined sugar or syrups to add taste to the food. This will make it even worse than the fat content. You should also avoid cookies, cracker, chips, wafers cakes and pastries as they all have high sugar or preservative content.

Junk Foods

Junk food is pretty self explanatory, its is nothing but junk. Junk foods are usually prepared poorly, fried, high in sugar and just cause overall poor health.

They have the most unhealthy kind of fat. The oil in which fast food is prepared becomes carcinogenic.

Alcohol

Alcohol is bad for your health and we all know it. It damages your liver and raises your cholesterol levels. However, one other thing that causes a serious problem is the sugar content. Alcohol is concentrated sugar that spikes your blood sugar levels, causing your insulin levels to get out of control. You must avoid consuming alcohol in large quantities. Your liver is one of the most important organs in your body and it performs more than 500 functions. Your liver takes 4-5 days in even recovering from mild consumption of alcohol.

Juices

Fruit juice may seem to be a natural and healthy option but it isn't. Fruit juice is a glass full of calories without any fiber to go with it. It will only spike your insulin levels and cause blood glucose management issues. If you want to have the nutrition of fruits, then eat them in their natural state or puree, but avoid drinking them as juice.

Chapter 14

KEY FACTORS IN THE SUCCESS OF INTERMITTENT FASTING

We have discussed at length the benefits intermittent fasting has to offer. It can be one of the best lifestyle changes you might have made to date. Intermittent fasting will make fat loss very easy and simple. Yet, intermittent fasting is simply not about weight loss. It is the key to holistic health. You can improve the overall quality of your life by adopting intermittent fasting.

Intermittent fasting can work as a stand-alone measure to good overall health. However, you can boost the advantages of intermittent fasting by incorporating some good thing like healthy and balanced food, exercise, and good sleep. Following the routine properly is also very important for the success and good results.

There are 4 Key Factors That Ensure Great Results Through Intermittent Fasting:

1) *Food*
2) *Exercise*
3) *Sleep*
4) *Routine*

Let's discuss them in detail.

Food

Food keeps us going and we need it for energy. You get all your nutrition from food and, therefore, you don't need to hold it back. The biggest problem with diet plans and calorie restrictive routines is that they may make you nutrient deficient. When you lower the calorie intake, you are also lowering the nutrient intake, and that can be bad for you're health.

Intermittent fasting is not much about what to eat and more about when to eat. The kind of foods you want to eat while following intermittent fasting will depend upon your end goals. If you want to lose weight then adopting a ketogenic diet that is high-fat and low-carb is ideal. Your focus should remain to reduce the number of meals you consume in a day and the time in which you consume them. Ideally, all your meals should be consumed within an eating window of 8 hours at the most. If you can reduce your eating window, it will be even better. Hunger is not a problem when you are following an intermittent fasting plan as your appetite will go down and your ghrelin release will adjust as per your eating schedule.

However, within those meals, you can treat yourself with a good amount of healthy food. You'll see that as you move ahead with intermittent fasting, you will feel less hungry and would still have all the energy.

If you are following a ketogenic diet for weight loss, then more than 70% of the calories should come from fats in your food. You should also try to eat healthy fats, get organic food, and include grass-fed meat or wild caught fish in your food. The next big item on your plate should be protein. It should be at least 20% of your diet as a low protein diet can lead to muscle loss. The least amount should be of carbohydrates. You should limit the carb intake to 5% and that should also come from fruits and starchy vegetables. Try ditching things like cakes, pastries, donuts, crackers, and bagels. Refined sugar or processed foods is a bad idea not only for weight loss but for your overall health too. There are many things that you can eat in unlimited quantities which you should try and consume . There are also lots of green leafy non-starchy vegetables. They do not add calories to your body, but are full of vitamins and minerals. Also they help make your meals nutrient dense and keep you healthy.

If you are wondering about the percentages of fat and protein, then there is no reason to worry. When you eat meat, you are not just eating protein but also fat aswell. The same goes for most of the foods. For instance, eggs have an equal amount of fat and protein which is ideal for healthy eating.

If weight loss is not what you are looking for and you simply want to adopt intermittent fasting for good health, then you do not need to watch your calories or fat-carb ratio. Simply keep in mind that fat, protein, and carbs all are equally important for your well being and all have their purpose. You must go for whole foods that are rich in nutrients and have a lot of fiber. It will keep your gut healthy and also provide the required nutrients.

However, one precaution you must always take and that is not to overeat. Many people feel that as they only have a limited number of hours and meals in a day, they should eat all they can to keep feeling full. It is a misconception. You would only end up feeling miserable due to overeating and may have digestion problems. Your hunger is not a result of your appetite but due to ghrelin release. Your hunger arises as per a fixed schedule if you have good eating habits. It means that even if you eat less, you would only feel really hungry at the time of your next meal. So, there is no need to stuff yourself.

Eating food rich in protein and fat will automatically keep you satisfied for very long as fat takes time to get processed. Eating a lot of fiber-rich food is also a very healthy way to keep hunger away and your digestion healthy.

Exercise

Exercise has a very important place in weight loss. If you want to lose weight, then your body is not going to burn calories without use. Exercise creates the demand for energy which your body fulfills by burning your fat. Therefore, exercise is crucial for burning fat fast. Intermittent fasting, however, increases the benefits of exercise for you. The insulin shortage created by intermittent fasting facilitates the production of HGH. It is very helpful in burning fat when you exercise. So, you can lose a lot of weight if you exercise in a fasted state while following intermittent fasting. Your metabolism increases and you can get slim faster. HGH also helps in muscle building, therefore, you would not only be losing belly fat but also gaining muscle. The best way to maximize the benefits of fat loss is to do high-intensity interval training. It creates a huge demand for energy and puts a lot of pressure on your adipose tissues or belly fat.

If you are already slim, then also doing aerobic exercises is very important. It keeps your muscles strong and your metabolism remains active. You will be able to maintain your weight and also remain free from most of the diseases.

Sleep

Sleep is very important for your health. Good sleep helps in the production of most of the helpful hormones. It also helps in keeping the feeling of hunger suppressed. Your stress levels remain stable if you are getting good sleep. So, sleep is very important and should never be ignored.

Some people feel that they do not require 7-8 hours of sleep and they can do away with less number of hours of sleep. They are making a mistake. Your body is a machine that needs time to repair and rejuvenate. When you are sleeping, your body is charging. You should let it recharge.

Sleep for better health benefits in intermittent fasting. If you are doing longer fasts, then you should try to sleep as much as you can. Sound sleep helps your body in the repair work, and it also increases the production of human growth hormone and ghrelin levels. However, it is important to make the distinction between sleeping and simply lying on the bed watching TV, or fiddling with your smartphone. The latter is a part of a sedentary lifestyle and has no positive impact on your health. On the contrary, it will only make weight loss difficult for you. You should always try to remain as active as possible in your awake time. Remaining active keeps your metabolism running.

Routine

Intermittent fasting is a lifestyle change. It is not some new fad weight loss measure. So, if you want to lose weight, remain healthy, and maintain a healthy weight, you must remain consistent with your routine. Following a routine is very important for the success and sustainability of the intermittent fasting program. Intermittent fasting is simple and there is no complication or complexity in it. However, it doesn't come with a timeline like most of the diets. You can remain healthy as long as you stick to the routine and therefore, consistency is important.

Another problem that people face is that they want a break from the routine at times. There is no technical issue in having cheat days as you can still maintain weight even if you have cheat days once in a while. However, the problem is that most people find it difficult to get back to the routine after they take a cheat day. The same goes for unhealthy eating. As we had discussed, most of the food items containing refined sugar or products like MSG are addictive in nature. They create cravings. Once you eat them, you would want to eat more and that could be a problem once you begin your intermittent fasting routine.

The best way to follow intermittent fasting is to follow a definite routine and remain consistent with it. This will pave the way to success for all your health goals.

Chapter 15

Important Points to Follow in Intermittent Fasting

Don't Overeat- It Will Only Make Things Difficult for You

You should always eat normally in your eating windows. Excessive eating will only make things difficult for you. By eating regular portions, you will not get energy deficient. Your body has a lot of fat to burn for compensating the energy deficit that you may face. Overeating will also cause digestion problems.

Exercise in Fasted State & Even on the Fasting Days

Exercise is going to make a huge difference in the speed of your weight loss. The more you exercise in the fasted state, the higher your fat loss would be.

The human growth hormone (HGH) production in your body is at its peak in your fasted state. You must work hard in the fasted state to fully utilize the benefits of growth hormone, it will give you the maximum fat burn.

You should never worry about stamina while working in the fasted state. Your muscles have an ample amount of glycogen to exercise and once glycogen stores are depleted, your body will start burning fat for energy. Burning fat has been the objective in the first place.

Drink Water and Remain Hydrated

A lot of detoxification takes place when you are fasting. To pass out all that waste, your body needs a lot of water. You must keep yourself hydrated at all times. If at any time you are feeling thirsty its important you take a drink. You should drink water on both fasting and non-fasting days.

Your body loses a lot of minerals along with water during this cleansing process. Add some sea salt and lime to your water. This will add some taste and also reduce the risk of stones. This would also replenish the loss of minerals through urination.

Water is a zero calorie drink. It also **suppresses your appetite** and, therefore, you should not have any fear of gaining calories through water. It will also help you in staying away from food for longer.

Drinking Unsweetened Black Tea or Coffee is Good

Tea and coffee have some antioxidants that help you in reducing oxidative stress and free radical damage. They are also natural hunger suppressors. So if you are feeling hungry, they'll help you. Tea and coffee also help you in cases like having a mild headache at the beginning of intermittent fasting or keto-adaptation. They do not add calories. However, do not overdo tea or coffee to suppress hunger. One or two cups a day should be fine.

Delay- Shift the First Meal of the Day Farthest

Delaying the first meal of the day is the best. The farther you shift it, the more your body gets the benefits of HGH and exercise.

Don't Fear Food

Most diets put a notion in the head of people that food and calories are bad for you creating a fear of food. It is the main source of nutrition. We still haven't adapted to producing energy through photosynthesis. There is no reason to fear food. The need is to understand food. Spend some time in understanding the food you eat. Select the right food for yourself that has all the nutrients. Focus on eating whole foods and organic foods. Eat as much green leafy vegetables as you can as they have lots of fiber, vitamins, minerals, and trace minerals. Avoid drinking your calories. Soda, alcohol, and sweetened beverages will simply add empty calories to your system. They will only spike the insulin levels in your blood. Avoid even fresh fruit juices as they add calories but have no fiber in them.

Chapter 16

COMMON MYTHS ABOUT INTERMITTENT FASTING

Intermittent fasting has emerged as a new trend. But, with it, many myths have also emerged that discourage people from adopting this lifestyle change. Intermittent fasting is a very safe and healthy practice. Myths regarding intermittent fasting are generally based on unsubstantiated assumptions and it is very important to understand their basic.

Some of the common myths regarding intermittent fasting are:

Myth #1: Morning Breakfast is the Most Important Meal of the Day

Food manufacturing companies have led us to believe that morning breakfast is the most important meal of the day. After all, they have hundreds of products to sell you for breakfast. You get repeated reminders through commercials that you must eat in the morning to remain healthy. It keeps your metabolism running, but this is just a lie. There is no doubt in the fact that the first meal of the day should be very healthy and should be the biggest meal of the day.

The reason is very simple. It is the meal you are going to have after prolonged fasting and it will replenish your energy stores. You must have a healthy first meal. It is also the meal that you'll be having while you have a productive day ahead with a lot of activity. This means that you'll have plenty of time to digest it properly. This makes it fit to have the biggest meal of the day at first and then start reducing the size of your subsequent meals so that your digestion keeps working fine.

However, there is no reason to have this meal early in the morning. Breakfast is the meal which you take to break your fast. It can be taken at any time of the day you feel fine. If your intermittent fasting schedule brings this meal to your lunchtime, then let it be. Do not play by the gimmick that morning breakfast is the most important meal of the day.

Myth #2: Fasting will Lead to Muscle Wasting

This is also a popular misconception that discourages people from any kind of fasting. First and foremost, eating doesn't lead to muscles. You gain muscles when you put them to work. Some of the muscle is lost, and stronger muscle replaces it. This is the simple process of bulking. Fasting or eating have no major role to play in it. While on any kind of fasting routine, your body produces a lot of growth hormone. This leads to faster fat burning and helps a lot in muscle bulking if you do high-intensity workout. Effectively, fasting will help in the building of muscles if you are doing the right amount of exercise and eating protein-rich food.

If you think that in absence of food your body will start burning muscles, then you are conceptually wrong. Your body has two main sources of energy namely carbohydrate and fat. When you eat food, the carbohydrate gets easily converted into glucose and your body loves to burn it. When you are in a prolonged fasting state, the carbohydrate supply stops and your body is forced to use the fat stores to produce the energy to run the body. Protein simply never comes into the picture. Burning protein is a cumbersome process. The body will only start eating itself when all sources of energy have depleted. An average person has enough fat to burn for a month if he or she goes without food. So, muscle wasting shouldn't be your concern if you are undertaking a planned fast, eating healthy and balanced meals, and doing exercise. Our ancestors had been living this way for thousands of years and they were fit, strong, and very active. They had to hunt and survive the odds, more so when they were out of food for long. Intermittent fasting wouldn't cause muscle wasting in general.

Myth #3: You will Get Weak if You Fast

This is a big worry in the minds of people. They are always afraid that they'll start feeling weak and energy deficient if they don't eat frequently. This book has so far made it clear that this is not the case. Your body has enough energy stored to keep you up and running for very much longer than a short interval of a few hours. You wouldn't feel weak even if you go without food for days as your body starts burning fat. In fact, you wouldn't even feel the hunger pangs after some time as your body gets adjusted to burning the fat stores.

The real thing to watch is the loss of some vitamins and minerals. When you undertake long fasts, your body loses some minerals in the detoxification process. Although you stop consuming food, you drink water and it comes out of your body with those minerals through urine. To prevent that, it is always good to have lime juice with a pinch of sea salt to replenish the lost minerals.

In intermittent fasting, there is no danger of nutrient deficiency as you are eating after a short interval daily. You can get all the nutrients, vitamins, and minerals through your meals. You'd neither feel energy deficient nor nutrient rinsed.

In the first few days of your beginning intermittent fasting, you can feel a bit weak and that's only because your body is adjusting to the fat burning process. There is no reason to get alarmed from it as it will go away within a couple of days and you'll feel more energetic.

Myth #4: You will have Low Blood Sugar

This is the big fear in the minds of people. They feel that the prolonged absence of food may result in low blood sugar. They will start feeling weak causing them to not being able to function properly. As stated above, this is a myth.

The feelings of weakness or dizziness, if at all, are temporary. Mostly, they are pseudo signs of hypoglycemia if the person is actually not suffering from type 1 diabetes. In general, insulin resistance is the reason for most of the problems. It lowers the ability of your body to absorb glucose in your bloodstream. Intermittent fasting effectively helps in reversing this condition.

However, you must consult your physician before undertaking any kind of fast if you are diabetic. Proper adjustment of your insulin levels will be required in that case. If you aren't already suffering from diabetes, dangers of low insulin levels with intermittent fasting are negligible.

For all those who are concerned that without the intake of glucose some of the most important functions of your body will stop, they are wrong. Your brain runs of glucose but it doesn't necessarily have to be supplied by the sugar you consume. Your body is a very well designed piece of machinery that can produce its required amount of glucose even by the oxidation of fat cells.

Myth #5: Your Body will Go into Starvation Mode

This is another popular myth that's based on ignorance. Short-term fasting or intermittent fasting will not send you into a starvation mode. A starvation mode is your body's defense mechanism to survive the longest even in the toughest conditions. In case, you stop getting food for long, your body will go into starvation mode and reduce the energy expenditure. It will lower your metabolism so that you can survive on your energy stores for long. However, this phase wouldn't kick in with intermittent fasting or even with fasts lasting 2-3 days. It is a survival mechanism that only kicks in real emergency situations.

In fact, several studies have proven that intermittent fasting increases your metabolism. It helps your body in becoming more active. Your reflexes get stronger and you are more attentive when you are in a fasted state. Your memory power and other cognitive functions improve considerably when you remain in the fasted state for a bit longer. This had been our body's natural response to stressed situations as it needed to be more focused to survive. So, you can take up intermittent fasting without the fear of lowering your metabolism at all.

Chapter 17

THE BEST THING ABOUT INTERMITTENT FASTING

Weight loss has become a global concern today. The increasing rates of obesity have put a large population at risk. Obesity comes along with a number of diseases and therefore, the concerns are even greater. There are a number of weight loss measures. The problem with almost all of them is that they are not easy and sustainable in the long run. This reduces their effectiveness and charm. Either it is dieting or a calorie restrictive regimen, and the possibility of following them for a long term is usually low. Apart from that, they stop showing results after the initial progress is made. If you are looking for quick gains, then you can try them but they aren't very effective in the long-run.

Exercise is a healthy and effective process. However, you will need to do a lot of exercise for a long period to get visible results. Without the help of healthy food habits, even the results from exercise will be low. If someone is already suffering from obesity then the chances of lowering the weight through exercise will significantly reduce. Moderate exercise is a good measure for maintaining the weight but for reducing the weight, you'll have to go all the way.

Yoga and aerobic exercises are also good health measures but they'll have little to slow impact on serious weight loss.

Intermittent fasting is a very good way not only to lose weight but also to keep yourself free from several lifestyle disorders.

Easy

It is very easy to follow a routine. You will simply need to follow your eating and fasting windows religiously and the rest will be taken care of by your body itself. Healthy food and exercise are very helpful in increasing the impact of intermittent fasting but it is also a great standalone measure.

Effective

Intermittent fasting is highly effective and tested method to lose weight. Its effectiveness has made it the favorite of people trying to lose weight or staying healthy. It is just not a weight loss measure but also a healthy lifestyle. You can stay free of a number of health issues by simply following intermittent fasting.

Convenient

It is one method that can be followed without the assistance of anyone in particular. You do not need to spend money or time on it. It reduces your expenses as your grocery bills and medical expenses start going down.

Chapter 18

INTERMITTENT FASTING IS FOR EVERYONE

Obesity and other health concerns are weighing down most of us. However, we fail to bring down the weight and make other corrections in our health due to several roadblocks. Diets, exercise, and other weight loss measures seem lucrative but don't seem to offer that ease. Intermittent fasting is completely different in this segment.

It is an easy and simple way to bring comprehensive health changes. You can follow intermittent fasting easily. Some of the major impediments that stop people from improving their health are:

Difficult Food Choices

Some people find it very difficult to follow health routines due to their food choices. Suppose you are vegetarian, then having an excuse to not indulge in rigorous exercise is always ready. People say that they cannot gather the stamina from their diet. It is no excuse, yet people make it. Intermittent fasting is a solution for you that you can follow easily irrespective of your food choices. Even if you are a vegetarian, nothing will stop you from intermittent fasting. You don't need to eat meat or eggs for getting the fat and protein. You can have vegetables, healthy fats like nuts, and other such things.

Wheat or Gluten Intolerance

People with an intolerance to specific types of foods like wheat or gluten also find it difficult to follow specific diet routines to lose weight. Intermittent fasting doesn't impose any restriction to eat any specific type of food. You are practically free to whatever you like as long as you follow the fasting windows.

Lack of Time

This is one of the biggest excuses given by people for not being fit. They always raise this excuse and say they can't find the time to get on the treadmill. Some people genuinely can't find the time to follow a specific routine. Intermittent fasting is a magic potion for such people. You can follow it without even wasting a single minute of your time. If you can exercise it would amplify the results but if you can't then you don't need to bother. The fasting period will do its job of burning the fat for you alone, and your health will improve significantly even if you do not do anything out of the ordinary and simply just follow the fasting routine.

Financial Constraints

There is no doubt in the fact that weight loss has emerged as an expensive affair. Diets, gym fees, pills, medication, and other measures cost a lot. The weight loss industry has become a $70 billion industry in the US alone. It requires you to spend money regularly, but many people can't find or simply don't have the money to spare on their health and end up being unhealthy.

If financial constraints have been stopping you from shedding the weight then intermittent fasting will work as a savior for you. It is absolutely free to follow. You don't need to spend a single dollar on anything, or need to buy any sort of kit or starter pack, or anything else that helps you in following the routine. Just simply, choose a plan that suits you and start following the fasting and eating protocols.

People Who are Always on the Move

Work can take you anywhere. If you remain busy and your work involves a lot of traveling then maintaining the membership of a gym can become tough. Such people also find it difficult to stick to a particular diet. Their schedules are erratic and life is always moving fast. However, even they can manage their weight effectively with the help of intermittent fasting. They will be able to lose weight even if they are not able to hit the gym on a regular basis. They only need to keep track of their fasting schedules and avoid eating excessive junk food.

People Who Detest Cooking

This includes plenty of us. In this hectic life, managing work pressures and cooking doesn't go along well. After a tiring day of work, cooking becomes a torture for many. However, it can't be worse than carrying pounds of fat on the body. Intermittent fasting can be followed even if you don't like cooking much. You don't have to follow a specific diet so you really don't need to cook daily. You can boil, grill or bake for the whole week at once. You can include a lot of vegetables and fruits in your diet. There are several ways to avoid cooking on a daily basis and still staying healthy. Intermittent fasting will help you in losing the weight.

Elderly

The elderly face a big problem in losing weight as their health doesn't permit them to engage in the strenuous physical activity. However, they can manage their weight much better with the help of intermittent fasting. In old age, the appetite usually starts to diminish.

The Different Factors That Make Intermittent Fasting So Successful are:

It is Possible for Everyone

Intermittent fasting is an easy way to remain healthy, and is possible for everyone. You can follow it irrespective of your age, gender or social and financial status. You do not need to stick to any specific thing while you are following intermittent fasting. There aren't many rules to follow so the chances of failure are few.

It is Flexible

It is one of the most flexible health routines to follow. There is no rigidity in rules. There is no binding on you to keep the fasts in day or night. You can follow any intermittent fasting method you like. If you want to go slow, no one is going to rush you. If you want to follow a tough regimen you can do so easily.

It Gives You Power and Control

Intermittent fasting gives you complete power and control. You do not have to go by the rules of anyone else. There is no peer pressure. There is no compulsion. You are free to follow it or have cheat days whenever you like.

It is the easiest way to stay healthy and fit. If health is your desire, then intermittent fasting can help you in the way you like.

Conclusion

Thanks for making it through to the end of this book. We hope it was informative and able to provide you with all of the tools you need to achieve your goals whatever they may be.

Intermittent fasting is an easy and effective way to bring a positive change to your health. It is a practice that can help you in losing weight and improving your overall health biomarkers.

This book has tried to explain the ways in which intermittent fasting leads to good health. The focus of the healthcare industry today is only on treating illnesses. Eliminating the root cause of the problems is something to which no one is actually paying any attention, and this is the reason for so many problems. Intermittent fasting, on the other hand, helps you in correcting the underlying causes of the problems.

You can enjoy a healthy and fulfilling life without compromising on anything if you follow intermittent fasting properly. This book has tried to put all the facts in front of you to be the better judge.

Good health is a treasure that should be preserved. Simply treating the illnesses is not the solution, you can only enjoy good health by eradicating the root cause of the problems.

This book has explained the science and essential knowledge behind intermittent fasting in a step-by-step manner and the ways it affects your health. It has also explained to you the ways in which you could get the maximum benefits from using intermittent fasting routines.

We hope that you will be able to benefit from this book and lead a healthy and fulfilling life.

Finally, if you found this book useful in any way, and have enjoyed this book, feel free to leave us a review. This will be greatly appreciated!

www.ingramcontent.com/pod-product-compliance
Lightning Source LLC
Chambersburg PA
CBHW020256030426
42336CB00010B/790